The Breakage Book

How to NOT Lose Your Hair!

By: Vaughn Leon

D1120831

Author Page

Vaughn Leon has over 25 years
experience in the field of cosmetology.
He's the Chief educator for Straight
Request products, since 1993. He has
trained and provided education at Trade
Shows and Seminars to audiences
exceeding 600 participants. A former
stylist of Southeast Bronner Brothers, Inc.
Dream Team. Vaughn has taught seminars
and classes nation-wide. Additionally,
Vaughn has produced over 25 videos
teaching how-to techniques for hair
stylists covering subjects of theory,
knowledge and technique, chemical
structure and hair color, coloring relaxed
and un-relaxed hair. Certified Master color
educator by Bobby J. Hunt of Color Elite,
in Orlando, Florida.

Dedication

This book dedicated to Jesus Christ, all my family, loved ones, friends and my mentors that not only believed in me, but stood by me in the tough times and encouraged me to keep moving forward. …the Hand that waters shall be watered.

-proverbs 11:25-

Contents

1

Hair Breakage and Hair Loss Epidemic

There is a billion-dollar market concerning hair loss. Probably rank in the top five things that men and women are worried about daily. Yet, the average person understands so little. I am sharing with you as a Master Edutainer (Entertaining Educator) but also as someone who cares about your hair and understand the value it is to your individual's self-esteem. There is an old saying, if your hair looks good, you feel good. In this book, we will review the why, what and how of hair loss. Understanding the fundamentals will help you to prevent hair damage. There are primarily two fundamental ways you lose your hair—hair loss and hair breakage.

To understand the fundamentals of these two types of hair loss, we will define how they work in simple terms. Hair breakage is external and deals with the strand itself, predominantly the part you see above the skin. Hair loss is internal, the section you can't see, dealing with the hair beneath the skin. But there are times when the two may cross paths. For instance, in reoccurring hair loss, chemical irritations or mild burns will cause hair loss due to damage done to the scalp while trying to relax the new growth. (More information in the chapter on chemicals).

There are a host of health issues that can result in hair loss: high blood pressure, the resulting medication for the management of thyroid problems, or vitamin deficiencies.

These are all contributors to malfunctioning—or in simpler terms, "broken"—glands that will cause you to lose hair from the scalp or skin. "Broken" means having been fractured or damaged and no longer in one piece or in working order.

According to Lisa Akbari of "World Trichology Institute" (2002), your scalp is your skin. It is important to always check what is going on with your body and your skin. Your skin is a constant reminder to you that your scalp is skin. The two are the same. Our body is a cohesive working machine, meaning that each part of our body is affected by what happens in another part of the body. Therefore, what is happening to your scalp-skin may be a result of what is happening in your body and may show symptoms on your skin at large. Because there are more hair follicles present on your scalp, the chances are greater that it will show symptoms of what else is happening elsewhere in your skin. Eczema is a great example of this effect of skin to scalp. Eczema is an extreme case of inflamed and dry skin.

The hair and skin are in the same family. They are connected like brothers and sisters. If one is affected by stress within the family structure, then most likely both may be affected. So, with this mind-set, it is important to keep the family happy and healthy.

Dehydration is a major stress component to hair breakage and loss. In simple terms, dehydration is the process of losing or removing water or moisture; it is a water or moisture deficiency. When the skin is dehydrated, the effects on the hair may not be detectable. If the skin becomes extremely dehydrated, like in the case of systemic lupus medication treatments, you might save more of the hair just by keeping the scalp properly clean and hydrated as much as possible. The first action you can take is to drink plenty of water. I know you have heard this many times before. It is true, but it's not the only thing. Many times have heard my clients say, "I drink my eight 8oz-glasses of water or more and my skin and scalp are still dry." Then I ask a few of these questions:

- "What do you eat?

    o Any fruits and vegetables regularly?

- Are you on any Meds?

- If so, do any of your Meds affect the skin, hair or nails?

- Do you have any health problems with you or in your family involve the Liver, Kidneys, Adrenals, Thyroid or Large & Small intestines?

These are all loaded questions, but the answers may reveal information that shows a significant effect on the skin, hair and nails. You will read about in future chapters and understand why. Improper diet is the second most important thing. Avoiding negatives, if you can, is third in this book. And later on in the book I will share with you some information on dietary foods, dietary supplements and things to avoid, to have the best skin, hair and nails your body can produce. Following these steps and making sure you are drinking the proper amount of water should hydrate your skin.

Shampoo regularly. Simply keeping the scalp clean and free from clogged pores can allow you to possibly keep more hair. The hair follicles can become clogged by debris and crust of the skin. If the hair cannot get through the hair follicle opening, it can contribute to scalp and hair loss problems such as alopecia. Alopecia means baldness, in simple terms.

Use great cleansers that are not drying to the scalp. If you have shampooed your scalp thoroughly and you notice that your scalp is flaking, it's most likely that the shampoo is dehydrating your scalp (the cleansers are too strong for your scalp), and it flakes because of the lack of moisture. If the scalp is properly cleaned, even with most dandruff conditions, it should not have flaking after cleansing. However, if you are dealing with constant discomfort and your flaking seems to keep getting worse please see a professional as soon as possible.

Use proper cleaning and hydrating shampoos. There are some good shampoos out on the market, such as carbon-focused shampoos containing different oils and natural cleansers to keep the scalp hydrated while treating the errors resulting from what you have done to your scalp directly or indirectly. Most problems are self-induced because you just did not know. Choosing to leave carbon-focused shampoos on for a long period may not be best for the hair shaft. It is best that after your last shampoo (especially after using a scalp treatment shampoo), you should use a hydrating shampoo to restore the hydration to the scalp and hair shaft. Hydrating shampoos should be designed to focus on hydration of the hair/scalp environment more than giving the hair strand more slip (a smooth feel) while shampooing. More slip is a play on the lack of knowledge on the one using the shampoo. But it sounds so good doesn't it; so does 2-in-1 shampoo, "Shampoo and condition at the same time!" My question is, can you add and subtract at the same time, No! You must do one or the other, first. I say, **"Clean the plate, then Hydrate!"** After that now your slip (smooth feeling) comes in, but it is from moisture conditioning.

Use hydrating scalp treatments. Even after shampooing is completed, it might be necessary for you to follow up with hydration scalp treatments. (We will address this later in a future chapter, and you will find the procedure at the back of the book.)

Avoid styles that would cause the scalp to dry out or remain unclean for long periods, such as up-dos and covering extensions. You might be wearing a protective hairstyle, but that protective hairstyle may not be conducive to a healthy scalp. The scalp may need to be shampooed often to prevent other things that only happen in a dehydrated state.

In the next chapter, we will go a little deeper into understanding the simple things most people overlook concerning hair and scalp/skin care because it just has not been introduced to them in this way or manner.

2

Understanding / the Structure of Hair, Skin, / and Their Relationship to One Another

Every process in hair care has a different but important hair/skin relationship. Let's start with the basics from the viewpoint of us here at Shear Techniques:

What Is Hair?
Any fine, threadlike strands growing from the skin of humans or mammals. Hair above the skin is dead. Hair is composed of three layers—cuticles, cortex, and medulla. We will only deal with two of the three.

Hair cuticles: These give strength and protection to the hair strand; they are like clear windows and lay like scales on a fish. Cracking or opening the cuticle can cause temporal or permanent change in the hair strand.

Hair cortex: This acts as the internal body, or the guts of the fish, all permanent color and texture change takes place here.

Other parts of the hair to be concerned with:

Hair bulb: The bulbous expansion at the base of the hair from which the hair shaft develops beneath the skin.

Hair follicle: The sheath of cells that surround the hair root.

Hair dermal papilla: A small nipple-like projection at the base of the hair root. It puts you in mind of the seed of plant from which a flower begins.

Hair shaft: The non-growing portion of the hair that protrudes from the skin.

HAIR ANATOMY

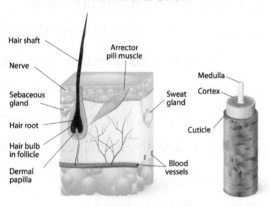

Hair shaft
Arrector pili muscle
Nerve
Medulla
Cortex
Sebaceous gland
Sweat gland
Hair root
Cuticle
Hair bulb in follicle
Dermal papilla
Blood vessels

What Is Skin?

Skin is the largest Organ of the body. Most people do not think of their skin as an actual organ. That's just skin, it's simply on the outside of the body holding everything in place. It is also called the integumentary system. It has intelligence, it breathes, and it lives. The skin regulates the temperature of the body. When it's cold it contracts to keep warm, but when it's hot it opens to cool down. Even the presence of odor, when sweating, is the body fighting bacteria that is present on the skin, and needs to be cleaned. Therefore, it truly lives! The hair and nails are its appendages, just like your arms and legs are appendages to the main body. Knowing this, you should start to treat and see it differently. In this section, we will deal with two of the three major layers of the skin (epidermis, dermis)

Epidermis, let's talk this through

What is the epidermis? It is the outermost part of the skin. It is made up of 5 thin layers. In some areas of the body only four are present. It does not contain any nerve endings within it, but the nerve endings sit just under the bottom layer. There are no blood vessels within the epidermis.–You cannot bleed until you go completely through all the layers and penetrate or scratch into the dermis.

What's the function of the epidermis? Waterproofing, keeping things consistent, protecting the body, and absorbing nutrients. (most of the body is waterproofed.) Twenty percent of its weight should be moisture. The presence of dehydration is either from external or internal imbalance (a disorder). If the skin is dry or dehydrated, it's damaged or has a disorder; because it is designed to hold 20% moisture within it.

There's always a disorder before disease. As a disorder advances, it goes into a diseased state. Warning comes before destruction. Are we listening? Do we know how to hear our body speak? Most of us do not listen or know how to hear it. In this busy world, we either run too much or have forgotten how to listen or were never taught how to. We all need to take classes on recognizing the signs. An industry mature Holistic or Trichologist doctor would be perfect to train you.

When you see a disorder, something that's not right, address it! Many things can be prevented by early detection; yes, it's true in hair breakage and hair loss also. There is ALWAYS a disorder before the disease state. The question is: do we respond when we see the disorder? When something looks out of order, check it out or stop what you are doing! If you're using a shampoo or doing a chemical service and something does not feel right and/or is not right, stop and rinse it off immediately.

If your skin is looking or feeling funny (not humorous), see doctor who specialize in skin disorder, holistic specialist, dermatologist, or other specialists of the body. If it is not an emergency, then you may want to start detoxing your body by drinking plenty of water until you can see someone. And start doing an Adventist or a more natural diet, and eat as much organic and non-GMO food as possible! (FYI. The body can start correcting itself during a detox; see the detox section after the conclusion.)

SKIN
LAYERS

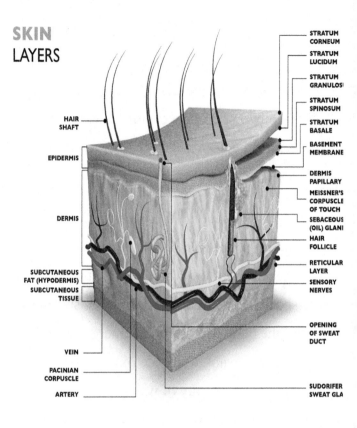

STRATUM CORNEUM

STRATUM LUCIDUM

STRATUM GRANULOS

STRATUM SPINOSUM

STRATUM BASALE

BASEMENT MEMBRANE

DERMIS PAPILLARY

MEISSNER'S CORPUSCLE OF TOUCH

SEBACEOUS (OIL) GLAND

HAIR FOLLICLE

RETICULAR LAYER

SENSORY NERVES

OPENING OF SWEAT DUCT

SUDORIFER SWEAT GLA

HAIR SHAFT

EPIDERMIS

DERMIS

SUBCUTANEOUS FAT (HYPODERMIS)

SUBCUTANEOUS TISSUE

VEIN

PACINIAN CORPUSCLE

ARTERY

Dermis

This is the middle structure of the skin. The main function of the dermis is to support the epidermis; there is an exchange of oxygen, nutrients, and waste products between these two layers.

What's in the dermis? Blood vessels, nerve endings, sweat glands, sebaceous glands (glands producing natural oil for your hair), hair follicles, hair roots, and dermal papillae. Blood vessels in the dermal papillae nourish all hair follicles and bring nutrients and oxygen to the lower layers of epidermal cells. Sebaceous glands are microscopic exocrine glands in the skin that secrete an oily or waxy matter, called sebum, to lubricate and waterproof the skin and hair of mammals. A hair follicle production occurs in these commonly known phases: Anagen (growth), Catagen (ending), and Telogen (resting).

1. *Anagen* — active growth phase (2–7 years) about 90 percent of your hair. Determines length.

2. *Catagen* — regressing, ending or also known as "**The Transition**" phase (10 days up to 3 weeks) about 1–2 percent of your hair is in this phase. Melanin production stops, the hair shrinks, the dermal papilla (hair seed, to make it a visual picture for you) detaches from the base, thus cutting off all nourishment gained through its blood supply.

3. *Telogen* — resting phase (3 months) about 10–14 percent of your hair. The life cycle is ending and beginning at the same time.

4. *Exogen* — shedding phase; independent of the first through the third phases, in which only one of seven hair strands might arise from a single follicle.

HAIR GROWTH CYCLE

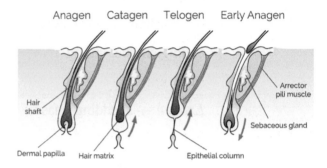

Anagen   Catagen   Telogen   Early Anagen

Arrector pili muscle

Hair shaft

Sebaceous gland

Dermal papilla   Hair matrix

Epithelial column

The Hair and Skin Connection.

Whatever you do to the hair strand root, the base above the skin, it will affect the scalp/skin. The things we do externally can have dramatic effects on our hair and skin. Here are some examples of style and chemical treatments and their negative results and basic remedies:

The External Factors
Relaxers

As you relax the hair you break down the epidermis, so use a base, and remember if it gets irritated the chemical has gone through or is going into the dermis. Weekly mild chemical burns can eventually cause hair loss.

Styles

For dry styles, pay attention to the scalp to make sure it is not dehydrated while trying to achieve your dry style.

Braids

Too tight and too much strand tension can pull out the matrix of the hair (dermal papilla) or cause you to pull it out during styling, like when pulling braids up into a ponytail. Too few strands used during braiding can cause the weight of the weave to pull it out from the root. With braids, do not wait for long periods of time between shampoos. Treat the hair and scalp in between shampooing. Use a good leave-in conditioner and dry shampoo, and use a proper scalp moisture product (look for products with natural ingredients). You do not want bacteria to build up on scalp or and infection to start. There was a news story where a mother left crochet braids in for 2-3 months without shampooing. A spider got into her hair and bedded down into her scalp. The spider laid eggs and couldn't be removed. That incident brought tears to my eyes and hurt my heart so much, but I use it to teach others about proper hair & scalp care regular cleaning.

Permanent curls

For dry curls- Shampoo and use rinse-out conditioner regularly. For wet curls- Shampoo and use a moisture retainer as needed. The first couple of days you have to use the activator heavier until you build up the moisture retention level. A wet curl will also help against dry scalp issues.

Bleach and color

Weekly mild chemical burns can eventually cause hair loss.

> *Bleach* – If the scalp is irritated with the lightener (bleach), remove and discontinue the bleaching process. Bleach has very little conditioner. It mostly deteriorates hair, hair color, and skin. Some conditioners are placed inside the bleach to use as an on-scalp bleach.

Demi-permanent and permanent color – If you are irritated by either of these products, it will most likely last for a short time before the irritation stops. However, that is still a sign that the dermis has been penetrated. Buyer beware!

Scalp treatments – If you are treating the scalp, the hair /scalp will probably need some type of rehydration after. They have two different levels of need in relation to how you want the finished style to appear. The hair need one level of hydration and the scalp needs another.

3

Awareness

Avoiding Skin Errors

Medicines

Medicines (Meds) are design to be a part of the healing process when our body is not functioning properly but they have some or major side effects that can also affect us in negative ways. However, it is said that the cure can sometimes be worse than the sickness. They have their place in our life and are necessary in many cases. In my opinion, as a society we are often too quick to "Go MEDs!" And I think that is mostly because the pharmaceutical companies control the airwaves and various communication avenues, specifically television. What you see and hear the most-you tend to migrate more sub-consciously.

In a sense, we are programed to medicate as a quick fix. Programing can work both for your good and for your bad. Therefore, the information that you might be receiving in this book, I hope that you will become a cynic and evaluate, read and review any information; and assess its potential good or bad for your health. If the medicine tells you that it affects the skin in any way, then it will affect your hair as well. If you have your hair relaxed, then that medicine may cause more drastic hair loss or breakage, because the hair has already lost about 70 percent of its strength.

Improper Shampoos for You

Over-the-counter shampoo may be wrong for your hair type, or too harsh for your scalp and dehydrate it, which can a cause a variety of problems. Not everyone can take that risk, especially people who already have sensitive skin or dry skin. A lot of people will be just fine. But if you want to be better than average result, "Go Pro!"

Major companies that sell directly to the public generally use cheaper and not as beneficial as professional product ingredients to get the job done. Generally, professional products will use a higher grade of products or ingredients for your hair and scalp that are generally more expensive but will perform better overall in the final outcome.

The Skin and Imbalances in the Body

First, remember this, a sensitive or dry scalp/skin is a damaged scalp/skin. There's something most likely on the inside that has your body out of balance. You might have to see someone in your circle of doctors (professionals). Here are a list of professionals and how they may be able help you.

A professional hairstylist. Considered your general hair doctor and probably your first line of defense, (other than yourself). Can perform basic to high level treatments for the hair and scalp. Assist in maintaining a healthy relationship between the two. One of the most important is to observe the hair and scalp for any abnormal occurrences. An educated hairstylist that you see on a regular basis or every 1 to 3 months for a hair checkup might notice un-normal imperfections in your hair, scalp/skin. Or somewhere else; such as arms, legs, face, lips or eyes (out of scope)? Then refer you to see a physician to find out more information so you can get examined and maintain the best health. An educated hairstylist can truly be part of your first line of defense to healthy hair, scalp and even health. They can create hairstyles to your pleasure.

A dermatologist. Dermatology is the branch of medicine dealing with the skin, nails, hair, and their related diseases. It is a specialization with both medical and surgical aspects. A dermatologist treats diseases, in the widest sense, and some cosmetic problems of the skin, scalp, hair, and nails. Thus, a skin specialist, but you should remember some problems are deeper than the skin. The skin may show or have problems, but those can be the result of something out of order on the inside causing the skin to be affected. Thus, "Deeper than the skin."

An endocrinologist. Endocrinology is the study of the medical aspects of hormones, including diseases and conditions associated with hormonal imbalance, damage to hormone glands, or the use of synthetic or natural hormonal drugs. An endocrinologist is a physician who specializes in the management of hormone conditions. For example, they can let you know about thyroids problems that can cause hair loss.

Your general physician. In the medical profession, a general practitioner (GP) is a medical doctor who treats acute and chronic illnesses and provides preventive care and health education to patients. According to the World Organization of Family Doctors (2014), They can also let you know to what degree a particular problem is and can refer you out to specialist that can examine even deeper to see if there is a problem you can not see without specialized test.

Holistic health doctor. A holistic doctor may use all forms of health care, from conventional medication to alternative therapies, to treat a patient. For example, when a person suffering from migraine headaches pays a visit to a holistic doctor, instead of depending solely on medications, the doctor will likely take a look at all the potential factors that may be causing the person's headaches, such as other health problems, diet and sleep habits, stress and personal problems... The treatment plan may involve drugs to relieve symptoms, but also lifestyle modifications to help prevent the headaches from recurring. They are also considered preventive specialist in my own and many others eyes. They will most of the time look outside the normal box of study and look for un-westernized methods of detection, such as iridology. Iridology is the diagnosis by examination of the iris of the eye. If you use it for nothing else but to detect an abnormality in a specific region is good all by itself. Then you can take that knowledge and see a doctor or specialist for more detail.

I have seen this to be very effective with other techniques combined. They also focus on herbs, prevention of illness, bringing the body into balance, and maintaining it. I myself have gotten it done. I was marveled at the accuracy about my "potential family weaknesses." They were "Spot ON" to say the least. From there I was told what to do to strengthen my body's systems so that I can live a now & later life without going through my elder kinsman's complications.

Trichologist (specialized hair loss doctor).
Trichology is the branch of medical and cosmetic study and practice concerned with the hair and scalp. Another definition is the study of hair and its diseases and how they relate to the scalp, according to Lisa Akbari

of World Trichology Institution. Trichology is a fairly new and untamed industry to the masses, but has been around a very long time. It is an extremely useful field. Someone who has studied Trichology and Licensed (or certified by the governing body) can also testify in court as an expert witness in dealing with hair loss. An example is in the Casey Anthony story in Orlando, Florida. The study of Trichology was used to find out if the child's hair loss on the duct tape around her head and mouth was lost before or after she had died.

Products and Process Can Help or Hurt

Shampoos and Products

Getting products that are mismatched with your hair's fabric type can cause minor to major shedding and breakage. A person with straight hair generally will have hair that tends to be more oily than other hair types. They need a shampoo that will get rid of the natural oil on their hair. They would use shampoos that may contain alcohol derivatives or that have a drying trait. For example, isopropyl or ethanol alcohols are considered to be short chain alcohol that are strong drying agents.

A loose wave or curly hair person will need something that is less aggressive on the drying or cleaning trait because they deal with a lesser amount of natural oil than a person with straight-hair. A person with over-curly to very tight curls deals with a dry hair situation. They don't need shampoo or conditioners counteracting the natural oils. They need shampoo that hydrates and moisturizes the hair strand.

From a Shear Techniques viewpoint, if we measured the hydration and moisture

that a person needs for their hair on a scale of 1 to 100 (percentage); i.e.,

> Straight hair
> 10–30% of hydration

> Wavy & loose curly
> 30–60% of hydration

> Over-curly & very tight curls
> 60–100% of hydration

If a person with curly hair uses a shampoo and conditioner that is perfect for a person of straight hair, it would not work well for their hair. Over time, even if they use great maintenance products, their hair can become excessively dehydrated and begin to shed and then break more aggressively the longer they keep using these products. Now, let's reverse the scenario. If a person with straight-hair person uses the perfect shampoo and conditioner for someone with over-curly and very tight curls, their hair will have a heavy, weighed-down, unwanted feeling, but it will not break, because hydration is present, even though it is more than desired.

If you have a tree next to a brook and one of its limbs falls to the ground, after a while the environment will get to it, and eventually you will be able to grab the branch and snap it with your bare hands. Now if one of the limbs falls into the brook, a hundred years could pass and you wouldn't be able to break it, because hydration is still present, even though it was separated from its life source of nutrients, the tree. **Dehydration is detrimental: Keeping hydration is essential!**

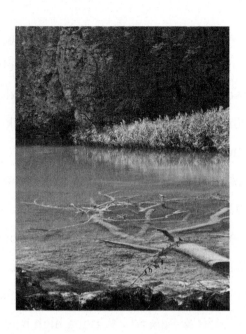

Heated Tools

Heated tools have quickly become one of the new ways to damage hair at home and sometimes in the salon. However, it is less likely in the salon because the stylists have more practice and more knowledge regarding the use of heated tools. Stylists find out the errors quickly and learn to stop before damage can occur (hopefully)! Plus, there are more people at home doing their own hair than there are people styling in the salon. In this fast-paced, do-it-yourself world we live in, manufacturers are doing direct sales and marketing phrases like "Use the same professional blow dryer & flatiron as your stylist, 450 degrees. Do it yourself!" (Hey, they have some great advertisements.) "And use our heat-protectant spray or serum with Moroccan or Argon oil. It comes free with three easy payments for your flat iron XK450 & Super-fast drying high heat blow dryer! Call now, and enjoy an evening out with lovely curls you did yourself. No more long hours in the salon waiting to get it done. Receive those same curls in minutes!" It is easy to get caught up.

It is great that you want to learn to do something for yourself, but you will not hear or see all of the "What had happened was...?" episodes, this usually means something went really wrong!, like in the famous YouTube viral video of the American teen burning her hair off. At least she made money out of her experience, I guess, but the average hair damage experience will *cost* you money to conceal your "I can do it myself" seizure! Like seizures, after a while you will stop and leave some things to the pros. See, what they don't say to people is what you don't know *can* hurt!

High-heated tools, especially ones at 450 degrees, are originally designed for the professionals. And now companies are making heated tools with one preset temperature of 450 degrees. A one-size-fits-all mind-set is dangerous. Many people don't know! But the companies know how to sell it. "Feel like a professional!" And everybody wants to feel like they can

_____! You can fill in the blanks yourself. Companies can easily reduce the temperature to a lower and safer one, but that doesn't go with the 450 degree sales and the marketing of "Like a Pro." You should get a tool with a temperature gauge. You should use a temperature that is easier to control so you will protect your hair from any thermal damage. If not, it might be best for you to see a professional you can afford. There are some who will work with you within your budget if you talk to them. Most pros can read and understand hair in its present state. Remember, the body and hair can change, so the amount of heat may need to change from time to time. The pros understand we all have different levels of hair thickness and porosity. Just knowing and understanding these two factors can help determine the proper amount of heat that should be used. My professional advice is to consult with the pro on what your hair needs. Do this at least once a month or every quarter (3 months).

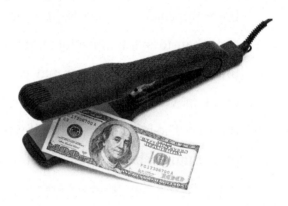

Avoiding Relaxer-Related Hair Loss and Breakage

You can have hair loss or breakage due to relaxer misuse. The issue at hand that can cause both is scalp burning. Let's look at the scalp first, because the degree of the burn can be the main culprit.

First-degree burns mean that fire or chemical has gone through the first layer of skin, the epidermis, at the top of the dermis. Some hair loss may occur. Hair bleach, color, and relaxer irritation is a first-degree burn. Repeated first-degree burns may cause some hair loss; too much too often with no time for the skin to recover may cause a problem. Give your skin a chance to recover. The body can heal itself with proper time in between treatments. Mild irritation is a sign from the body's nerve endings to stop the treatment before it goes any further. Don't ignore this sign! You are still in a safe zone (see image).

Second-degree burns mean the substance has gone past the epidermis down into around 50 percent of the dermis, where the hair bulb lives. About 50 percent hair loss may occur (see image).

In third-degree burns, the substance has gone down to the base of the dermis, resulting in permanent hair loss and destruction of blood vessels (see image).

For example, in the case of a famous pop star, Michael Jackson (reported in the Daily News in January 27,1984, http://www.huffingtonpost.co.uk/2014/01/27/michael-jackson-burnt-scalp-pepsi-drugs-dependence-death_n_4674169.html) was said to have had second- and third-degree burns on his scalp during a soda commercial accident. He received scalp burns from his hair catching on fire. A report came out before his death that they could grow new hair from this region. You cannot grow hair where there are no blood vessels or dermal papillae present. I wager you that this was a lie.

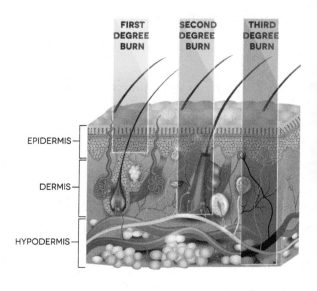

FIRST DEGREE BURN   SECOND DEGREE BURN   THIRD DEGREE BURN

EPIDERMIS—

DERMIS—

HYPODERMIS—

Now let's look at hair strand breakage. There are a few keys to getting hair relaxing correct: **Know Your Hair, Know Your Product!** Sounds familiar, doesn't it? What type of hair fabric do you have? Straight, wavy to loose curl, or over-curly to very tight curls? Now remember each fabric's characteristics. This will tell you what can be done safely with your choice of relaxer. Your next step is to know your product and its effect on the hair. What do you want out of relaxing your hair, and what kind of relaxing fits you? Let's look at the four forms of relaxing.

1. **Softening the hair fabric** – No physical change. Softening the cuticles to receive product and allowing the hair to be easier to manage. Can be done on all fabrics of hair. It takes about 1-3min to do. All times are relative to the client's texture, porosity and/or using a professional eye & knowledge of product.

2. **Texturizing the fabric** – Where 30–60 percent of hair texture is change or removed. Not for straight-fabric hair. Opens curls, but not to the point that it's too straight. This will at

most times be enough for wavy to loose-curl hair. Should take about 3-5 minutes, some clients will need a little smoothing. All times are relative to the client's texture, porosity and/or using a professional eye & knowledge of product.

3. **Relaxing the fabric (level 1) –** Where 60–85 percent texture change or removed, for wavy to over-curly hair fabric. This is the national standard for relaxed straight. This works best for people living in northern areas. My advice on Levels 1 & 2 use manufactures instruction for times and procedure: unless guided by a licensed & trained pro.

4. **Relaxing the fabric (level 2) –** Where 85–95 percent texture change or removed. This is generally for

very tightly curled fabric hair. Best for southern tropical regions, because of the amount of moisture in the air.

For professional hairstylists, consultation with the client is a must, especially before doing chemical and mechanical service and before every client, each visit. You need to be informed as much as possible of your clients' hair and scalp history. There are some great consultation forms that you can get online. (See free consultation at the back of book). Also visit: http://www.insuringstyle.com/wp-content/uploads/Hairstylist_Client_Consultation_with_Weave.pdf.

Basing

We the professionals must start with the
standard of protecting our patron or client:
being prepared and protecting the skin! This
is called basing the scalp. Basing is the
technique of coating the scalp with a
protective product that probably has a
petroleum base and has other products in it
that benefit the skin; like an oil to add
moisture and aloe to promote healing. In
standard basing, you will part the hair into
four large sections. Then you will create
subsections and place it on the entire scalp.
Basing may not be considered a necessary
step to some, but it should be. No one that
comes in for a relaxer wants to leave with an
unfinished relaxer with his or her scalp
severely burned.

This is important also for legal reasons. A salon and the professional can be sued and lose the case if they have not done everything in their power, as a professional and as a salon owner, to protect their client. Client protection and protecting the scalp is a must for the best service. They should remember that a sensitive scalp is a damaged scalp—this actually means the epidermis is not holding its proper weight in moisture. Something external or internal is affecting it. It is also important to rehydrate sensitive and non-sensitive scalps before relaxing by properly basing the scalp; the basing process creates a protective barrier to help prevent from irritation. If you notice that your client's scalp is dehydrated, or because your client has irritated their scalp from wearing hat to scratching it, you might want to let the base sit 10 to 15 minutes to absorb into the scalp and rehydrate it for maximum protection. This will give you added protection from the chemicals.

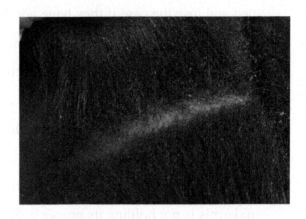

Scalp before basing

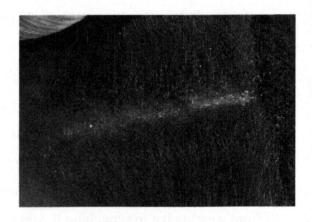

Base applied

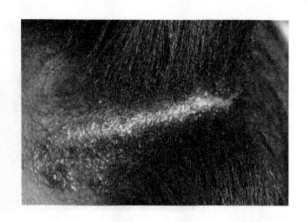

How the scalp should look after base

has been smoothed on the skin

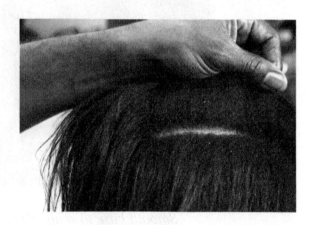

Open parting to prepare subsection

for basing

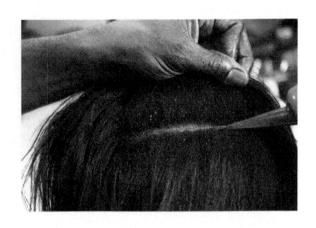

Apply base to scalp Only

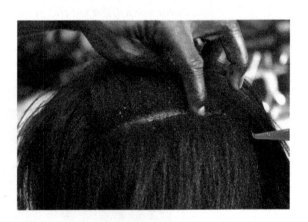

Smooth base to scalp/skin

Chemical Relaxers

There are more than two kinds of basic
chemical relaxers, but let's deal with the

two most popular in Northern America:
sodium hydroxide and calcium hydroxide
(sensitive scalp, Guanidine relaxer).

Sodium Hydroxide

It is known as the best relaxer, mostly
because it has a clean application, meaning
it leaves no residue behind on the hair.
Some say it's better for the hair but harsher
on the scalp! I say this is partly true. It may
be better for the hair as long as the hair
doesn't have what Shear Techniques calls
color, which is any color, or pigment, that
you change to from the natural **or present**
color level, **to** any higher color level **that**
you lift to with a 20-vol. (or higher)
developer. To color on sodium hydroxide–
relaxed hair, you should use a nonpermanent
color, an according to state boards across
the nation. This may not be true in all
situations. You can use some permanent

color on permanently relaxed hair, but use extreme caution (let a professional do it). To stay on the same level, lower it, or to add a hue, we recommend you mostly use an opaque or translucent demi-permanent or semi-permanent color. The US national licensing says not to use sodium relaxers on color-treated hair. I say follow the US national licensing because of all the negatives associated with sodium hydroxide relaxers, despite it being labeled as the number 1 relaxer for its clean application.

Here are a few negatives of using sodium relaxers:

1. It is easier to over process
2. Creates the potential for poor application from rushing
3. Irritates the scalp fast.

Calcium Hydroxide

Calcium hydroxide relaxers are normally slower moving than sodium ones. Some say they're easier on the scalp and harsher on the hair strand, mostly because the compound has a larger molecule and it leaves a calcium residue. With today's arsenal of shampoos and conditioners that remove the calcium residue the same day it is applied, that cannot really be considered a negative any more. I would say that this makes it the better choice for high-lift colors. Remember, according to the state board licensing, it is not recommended to use sodium hydroxide relaxers on permanent color-treated hair—calcium hydroxide is somewhat the opposite of its sodium counterpart.

Some positives of using calcium relaxers:

1. It's slower to over-process,

2. Allows more time for correct application,

3. It is also slower to irritate the scalp.

The thing to remember is: just because it's not irritated, that doesn't mean it's not working. When relaxing hair, people tend to relate burning to the stopping point. True, it is a stopping point. But do not look for the burn before you stop, because it is not supposed to burn if you base the scalp properly and with proper application. Look at the new growth to judge, NOT the irritation. People, stylists included, tend to wait for the burn when they should be learning to read the hair during the process instead. You cannot read it unless you are looking at it and checking it. And that can't be done from across the room. Relaxing hair with too strong a product is another problem. It is a complex process and the damage **can't always** be seen immediately; sometimes the damage is not seen until the hair begins to shed more than normal days or even weeks later. At this point, there is a loss of the hair fabric's *elasticity*—this is the hair strand's ability to stretch and return. It could also be a sign that the cuticle is opened too much. Once you have straightened the hair to the desired straightness, stop and rinse. Allowing the relaxer to continue to sit will, quote, "relaxed it too hard." You are removing more of its strength than needed, thus opening the cuticle even more. If you desire to ever have a high-lift color, then this is a definite no-no. Once a high-lift color is applied, the truth about your unhealthy hair-relaxing will be shown even more.

Traditional Keratin Relaxing (Formaldehyde base product)

Let's define this as a straightening method where the natural pattern does not return after shampooing in a single sitting but remains straight until the product has worn off. This could take months or even a year of shampooing, depending on how often shampoo is used. Some people shampoo daily, or three times a week, and some shampoo every week or two. Most manufacturers of this product tell you that keratin treatments last about 36 shampoo sessions; this is 2 to 3 shampoos a session. . This was based on the time it would take for the formaldehyde treatment to wear off the hair and to see the texture return.

Basically, you merely need to have the correct hair fabric and texture to use it safely. Best used on oily hair types. This type of relaxing is temporary but can have breakage issues down the road on hair that has a dry natural state. The process creates a type of lamination over the hair strand. This is why you don't see a return of the natural curl pattern until the product has worn off a bit. During this period, no external moisture treatments can get into the hair strand. This, coupled with high-heat tool usage, such as flat ironing and roller-brushing techniques, can cause extreme dehydration to the hair strand. Then you might see dehydrated hair strand breakage because there's no elasticity left. On the other hand, hair with an oily natural state can handle the traditional keratin treatment and suffer no breakage or dehydration. Therefore, the important factor in all hair-straightening process is to **know your hair fabric and know your product.**

Shampooing a traditional keratin treatment that lasts for 36 shampoos:

Daily = 5+ weeks, or 1 month and 1 week (straight hair)

Three times a week = 12 weeks, or 3 months (straight, loose wave, or curly hair)

Once a week = 9 months (loose wave or curl, over-curl, and very tight curl)

Every other week = 18 months (over-curl, and very tight curl)

(Every 3 months of new growth needs a treatment procedure on the new growth section, but not necessarily on the hair strands already treated.)

Why do some hair smoothing products expose me to formaldehyde?

Many keratin-based hair smoothing products contain formaldehyde dissolved (and chemically reacted) in water and other ingredients in the product. Because of the way the formaldehyde reacts in these products, some manufacturers, importers, or distributors might list other names for formaldehyde on product information or might claim that the product is "formaldehyde-free." Formaldehyde might be listed as methylene glycol, formalin, methylene oxide, paraform, formic aldehyde, methanal, oxomethane, oxymethylene, or CAS Number 50-00-0. All of these are names for formaldehyde under OSHA's Formaldehyde standard. There are also chemicals, such as timonacic acid (also called thiazolidinecarboxylic acid) that can release formaldehyde under certain conditions, such as those present during the hair smoothing treatment process. The bottom line is that formaldehyde can be released from hair smoothing products that list any of these names on the label and workers can breathe it in or absorb it through their skin. Workers can be exposed to formaldehyde during the entire hair straightening process, especially when heat is applied (e.g. blow-drying, flat ironing). https://www.osha.gov/SLTC/formaldehyde/hazard_alert.html

Again, know your hair, know your product.

Smoothing Systems (Non-Formaldehyde base products)

Let's define this temporary relaxing system. It's like a perfect thermal press technique. The hair strand remains straight until shampooed, or until exposed to an environment with heavy humidity, or submerged in moisture. Beware of long hot showers! Then the natural hair pattern will return. This smoothing procedure elongates the hair's pattern, refortifies the inner bonds to hold its temporal straight shape longer, and reduces hair frizz. Every time you reheat the treated hair, it reactivates the active agent, the carbon cysteine bond **is an example of a key ingredient used for smoothing systems,** to shrink the thickness of the strand and straighten the hair.

Apply correctly. Be sure you are applying correctly. If your hair doesn't hold its straightness then it might not have been sealed into the hair correctly. This can be due to not enough product applied, or the hair being flat ironed too quickly during the sealing process to adhere to the hair. This is easy to fix. Reapply and flatiron slower to seal the product in properly. The reason why most of the companies instruct you to use a small, fine-tooth comb is because they want a complete distribution of the product over the entire hair strand. And nothing gives you a better sense of the distribution than a fine-tooth comb.

Don't overuse your heat tools. Don't use the wrong amount of heat for your hair type. The hair fabric and thickness matters. Thick straight hair fabric can take a lot of heat, as much as the other hair types of the same thickness. The thinner the hair type, the lesser heat you must use compared to the thicker of the same fabric type. Don't try to make it straight with the heat tool; let the product do its job. Going over the hair strand too many times, or with too high of a heat for the hair strand, can cause heat damage. Then your hair will have thermal damage and won't return to its natural curl pattern. Learn to read the hair strand for proper hair care!

If you feel the flatiron, thermal iron or blow dryer is going into the hair too quickly, or the hair strand is giving in to your thermal tool too easily, then it's

probably too hot for that strand of hair.
Again: know your hair, know your
product—in this case, your thermal tool
being your product.

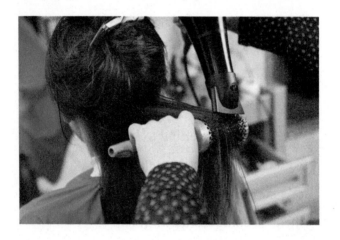

Avoiding Color Breakage

Coloring is the hair industry's biggest money maker. To understand why hair breaks in coloring or becomes damaged, you first must understand how the product works. Everything starts with knowing your hair and knowing your product. This section begins with knowing the product, because by now you are getting to know your hair from the previous chapters. So first of all, let's simplify hair coloring with a few of Shear Techniques definitions:

Basic tint – Depositing color pigment on the same level or lower to alter its surface color without changing its permanent pigment. This is done with rinses, semi-permanent, and demi-permanent color.

Coloring. *Altering the present permanent pigment to a higher level, a brighter color.*

This will make it easier for some to understand. The two most important forms of hair coloring in this section are bleaching and permanent coloring.

Permanent tint – Depositing color pigment on the same level or lower to alter its permanent color. This can only be done with Permanent color or a toner (which is actually permanent color with no lifting ability. **(Shear Techniques Permanent Color definition has a slightly different definition; given under color types)**

Color Types

Rinse – surface tint that lasts from shampoo to shampoo. Cannot cause any breakage.

Semi-permanent – Surface tint that lasts for 4–6 shampoos. Cannot cause any breakage.

Direct dye semi-permanent – lasts the same amount of time as semi-permanent, but stains the cuticle, and the stain remains after the pigment is gone.

With rinses and semi-permanent you only have to worry if you have an allergic reaction or not, this is rare, or maybe not because of all of the low preforming immune issues.

Demi-permanent – Surface color lasting 4–6 weeks or from chemical to chemical, such as bleach, relaxer, and permanent color. It doesn't change the hair's present permanent pigment, but it does lift the cuticle and barely penetrates the hair to make the tint last longer. The coloring substance has a larger molecule than in permanent coloring. It comes in two forms; both are great when you can use them. An activator is needed with this product.

1. **Translucent demi-color** – Allows light to pass through and illuminate the pigment; semitransparent. This tint is gentler than the opaque Demi-permanent. Very little chance for any hair breakage. I recommend this one on fine-coarse hair; and even on the same day as a relaxer. If the hair is very thick and

healthy, you might want to bump up to the next choice.

2. **Opaque demi-color –** Not able to be seen through, a dense color. It reflects light; not transparent. Can cause some delayed breakage if the hair is not healthy enough to handle it on the same day as of a relaxer treatment. I don't recommend it on most fine or weak hair the same day as a relaxer. The hair needs to be in a truly healthy state and with a medium-

coarse nature or thicker. This particular demi-color is more aggressive than its counterpart, translucent demi-color.

Permanent color – Lifts and diffuses the present pigment and deposits a new color base while conditioning slightly. This happens during the processing time, called the oxidation period. When the lifting action stops, around the last 10 minutes of the oxidation period, the majority of the color deposits in. This is known as the "drop and swell" phase. This is about 70–80 percent of your new color base foundation. You must use a developer to trigger the permanent color to work. Permanent color has a smaller molecule, than rinses, semi and demi-permanent colors, to penetrate into the cortex and change it. It comes in translucent and opaque as well. With today's advanced formulas, permanent colors are used as demi, permanent, and toners. This action is controlled by the choice of the developers and is best done by professionals.

Toner – falls on the side of a Shear Techniques tint category. It has no lifting action involved, even though it is a permanent color. It normally only takes 2–10 minutes, but if you leave it for the full 10minutes it will get darker than your target level (I recommend this as a professional only procedure to get your target color more defined).

Lighteners/bleach – Lighteners lift and dissolve the present pigment of the hair. You have on- and off-scalp lighteners. Adding in some conditioners makes it an on-scalp version. Lighteners are very harsh on the hair and have few conditioners. Their main purpose is to lift and erase; DON'T FORGET THIS! We may tweak, buffer, and/or add color to it, but the main purpose of lighteners is to lift and dissolve. So many companies are adding color, but this is good marketing stuff, **so be Careful!** It's not permanent color. When you have gone too far, Shear Techniques calls this form of lightening *bleaching*; you've performed the wrong process for that head of hair to be healthy. You've either lifted too much or did it too fast to control. I've seen so many use plain and specially colored lighteners and bleach the hair real high and then put on an artistic color, vibrant semi-permanent, and love it, not knowing the hair is more than DEAD now and sooner or later must be cut off or watched as it breaks off all by itself. This is the harshest product to use on hair and may affect the scalp also. So be mindful and watch for the signs to stop!

Now let's talk about some of the color problems that occur in a few situations:

1. Bleaching untreated hair-

    a. Simple bleaching, untreated hair normally doesn't give you a problem concerning breakage. But you might have a problem hitting your target color or level. This normally comes from knowing the hair that you're bleaching, classes, and experience. Just follow the directions. The problem comes with going too far and too long. Bleach is a keep your eye on the product. If you plan on doing more than one application and you want what you want, see a professional, Not YouTube

University. That could turn out to be a hit or miss!

2. Coloring relaxed hair-

   a. One-step permanent coloring on healthy relaxed hair should be perfectly fine. Even if you use 40 volume developer. Normally where the problem comes in is what people do NEXT! Then they blame it on the color. If it hasn't started breaking and shedding that day or the next, you're fine. Just use the proper shampoo and conditioner for your hair fabric, use a heat protectant, and turn those hot tools DOWN. Notice these are the same instruction for uncolored hair. **Know your hair, know your product.**

      i. Toners- I hold toners in the one-step category. But you normally use it after a prior step, after lighteners or permanent color. It's used to fine tone the desired color on whatever the present level. Because it only sits for such a short time. It's safe on it's own.

ii. Rinses and semi-permanent are even safer. Squirt, brush or glob it on. Add heat for desired time and rinse. Just be careful with your pretty pillow case, clothes and getting caught in the rain (It might not match your blush as it runs down your cheek)

b. The Relaxer before and after a color are pretty much the same.

c. Control your product- If you only have half and inch of new growth, then your product shouldn't be 3-4 inches or more down the hair shaft. *(see image below)*

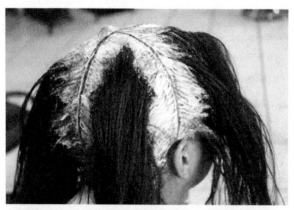

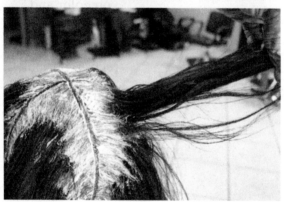

(This client had 1.5 inches of new growth. Notice the relaxer stops shortly after the new growth)

       i.   Don't relax the hair so hard. This will take away more of the strength of the hair then needed. When the hair gets to the straightness that you desired, rinse immediately. Don't wait for the burn. It's not suppose to.

          1.   Relax safely- wait 2-3 weeks after you color and condition it every week before you relax if possible

3. Bleaching Relaxed hair-

   a. Let a PRO do it! See the instructions given for proper lightening aren't for relaxed hair. Save Yourself from being a YouTube horror flick... or even on "Right This Minute!!!"

4. Coloring Thio hair (perm and dry or wet curls)

    a. This could be tricky too. If you're going dark ok, but going lighter; See a Pro! The little things can make a difference and can make things tragic.

5. Wrong person for color

    a. If a person is someone that doesn't take care of their hair, one step coloring is best. Leave the super high-lift and advance coloring for someone that will be a walking model of your work; even if you're the stylist and model.

Too Much Too Soon

In this crazy world, today, no one wants to wait for anything! That's why we get caught up in some marketing ads:

"You don't have to wait. Buy this tool now and do it at home yourself."

"Why wait for a permanent color to process its full time when you can use our color bleach? It works fast!"

"Relax and get a permanent color the same day!"

What you are not being told is that by not waiting there might be consequences and repercussions: You can burn out your hair because you have no idea how to read your hair like a pro.

You might over-bleach your hair because you are looking at the vibrancy of the depositing color, rather than reading the pigment level. Your hair will open like the branch on the ground. Now your hair is extremely dehydrated and you may need major weekly conditioners just to keep your hair on your head until you grow a new head of hair over the next 1.5 years or so. You'll be in your stylist's chair spending lots of money every week because you have to get professional conditioning.

I'm not saying these quick tricks and skills can't be done by a pro. A professional might do all of them, though this is not recommended. I just want you to be knowledgeable of the risks so you don't break your hair off.

When we do chemical services on our head we break down the chemical structure of our hair and skin. Sometimes one of the best things is proper R & R (rest & relaxation), sometimes even from all chemicals. Yes, I'm talking about for your hair and skin too. Give the hair and your skin proper rest and conditioning between services. Even if you're not a regular salon person. Go in and pay for an inexpensive consultation. It's like the deductible you pay for when you go and see your physician about your body. A hairstylist can be thought of in the same manner. Then purchase what you need from them, instead of buying something that your stylist doesn't know as well as the products he/she uses. You would want your doctor to prescribe a drug or product that he knows and can tell you all about. Wouldn't you? So fill your hair prescription right there! Also, the better you eat the stronger everything gets. The better your diet, the stronger hair strand you produce, and the healthier your skin will become. The hair gets its nutrients and strength from the blood. So if you're having troubles from beneath the skin, go see someone who specializes in that area. Don't be surprised if the first thing they recommend for you to do is to detox your

body. I think sometimes the first and best
thing to start off with is getting the bad out.

4

Keep Hydrated

Know What True Hydration Is

What's the difference between moisture and hydration? That's the elephant-in-the-closet question. But both help the hair and skin's elasticity, the ability to stretch and return to normal.

Hydration involves a small water molecule that creates an internal balance of fluids. Humectants are used to draw in water. Simply put, it is moisture (water) on the inside. Moisture is a larger molecule and sits on the surface. It is water and conditioning on the outside. As related to hair, it gives your hair the ability to stretch and return to its normal position. A lack of moisture will break off as you comb your hair in the morning as you get ready for work because it's too dry to give way to styling your hair.

With that said, remember the story about the tree limb and the brook to help you understand the importance of keeping your hair and skin hydration in check. We are made up of mostly water, so we understand that water is life!

Remember our story:

Imagine you have a tree next to a brook, and a limb breaks from the tree and falls to the ground; the environment can get into the limb and affect it. Over time, it will lose its hydration and moisture, then dry it out! Eventually, I can walk over and crush the limb easily with my bare hands. If another branch falls off the same tree but into the water, it could sit in the brook for a hundred years, and if I take it out of the water I would have trouble breaking it because hydration and moisture are still present!

Even if you don't have the correct hydration and moisturizer for your hair at home to achieve a certain style you want, and your hair is dry or brittle from bad coloring, bleaching, thermal tools and/or relaxing, technically you can go heavy on hydration and moisture to keep your hair from falling out until you can see a professional and buy the best products for you. When you have a lack of water greater problems comes because of the dry state. Just like cirrhosis of the liver by way of alcohol (the alcohol has a drying, dehydrating, trait), the liver becomes dehydrated with scar tissue and unable to function properly. Now you will have skin issues. **Remember, dehydration is detrimental. Keeping hydration is essential.** Think about how much life lives in the rain forest… (take a second and see it in your mind.) Now, think about the little bit of life in a desert. Now think about the abundance of life in a rain forest. Drinking water is not the only way to keep the body hydrated. What you eat is the second major way. If you eat an acidic diet your body won't have the proper nutritional based hydration. Your body should be slightly alkaline, 7.4-8pH is Healthy level. A western diet is normally very acidic with the hamburgers, pizza, French fries and various fast foods, but that's for the next chapter. You can get part of your water for life through your food (that's why juicing has become so big for health) Water is LIFE!

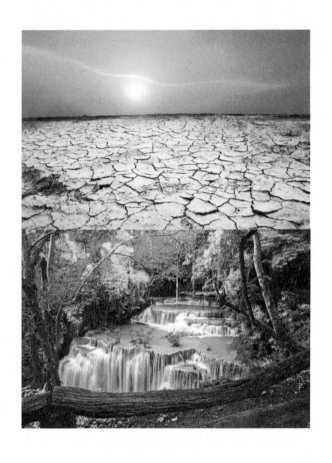

Please look over my pH scale for your own Knowledge.

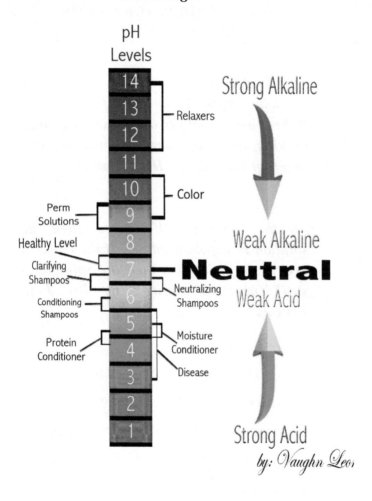

pH Levels

Strong Alkaline

14
13 — Relaxers
12
11
10 — Color
9 — Perm Solutions
8 — Healthy Level
7 — Clarifying Shampoos
Neutral
6 — Conditioning Shampoos / Neutralizing Shampoos
Weak Acid
5
4 — Protein Conditioner / Moisture Conditioner
3 — Disease
2
1

Weak Alkaline

Strong Acid

by: Vaughn Leo

95

5

Deeper Than the Skin:
Things you can do

*"Let food be thy
medicine and medicine be thy food."
"There are in fact two things, science and
opinion; the former begets knowledge, the
latter ignorance." By Hippocrates*

*"If the cause is self-induced, then the
solution is self-induced too. If the cause is
toxicity & deficiency, then the solution is
sufficiency and purity." By Dr. John
Bergman*

This chapter is designed to help you be proactive in what to do to prevent breakage. This knowledge is based on a compilation of my 30 years of experience and my study of hair loss and breakage.

There is one reoccurring element that shows up as an underlying cause in the background though out my research. It is the deteriorating health issues and resistant levels of a client's skin and hair. As I continued to serve my clientele and teach others, I developed an urgent need to find answers to the question of a cause and effect relationship between unhealthy hair and unhealthy skin. I began and became even more of a lateral and a critical thinker. I took color classes to grow my knowledge only to see that there were even more problems and I had more questions, but I could now answer more of them than before. After mastering many things in the color field and educating others, I dove deep. I studied ingredients, procedures and into the field of Trichology. Then started taking classes in Trichology, after that, again studying health issues resulting in skin problems and hair loss. This chapter is to share the connection that I found with my knowledge of being an educator since 1993 and all the knowledge gained from classes and sitting with masters of hair and color.

Baldness goes deeper than the skin. Technically called Alopecia, baldness is partial hair loss or the complete absence of hair from areas of the body where it normally grows. Specifically, Alopecia Areata (AA) is an autoimmune disease. Autoimmune means that the body's immune system attacks the body. In AA, the body attacks its own hair follicles, causing you to lose your hair. Most forms of Alopecia are from an immune issue.

"A careful history and examination of shed hairs will reveal the etiology *(the reason for)* **of most alopecias due to systemic processes. Telogen effluvium** *(a* *scalp disorder characterized by the thinning or shedding of hair...)* **is preceded by a severe systemic stress** *(stress within your body's system)* **occurring at least two months prior to the loss of normal club hairs. Most other causes involve damage to the hair follicle, which leads to the shedding of dystrophic, brittle anagen hairs. A history of drug ingestion** *(mostly medications)* **and nutritional compromise** *(bad diet)* **or concurrent symptoms** *(combination of two or more problems at the same time)* **suggest a genetic, endocrinologic** *(endocrine glands & hormones)***, collagen vascular** *(a connective tissue disease)* **or infectious etiology will lead to an acute** *(severe)* **diagnosis."**

By Dermatologic clinics

To put it in simple terms, the reason for most baldness problems is shedding hair and an internal system error of the body attacking itself, resulting in alopecia. The error is caused by stress within the body within 2 months prior to the loss of hair. The majority of the other causes comes from damage to the hair, which leads to bad shedding and the hair becoming brittle while in the growing phase of the hair cycle. A history of medications that impair the internal systems of the body, a nutritionally-deficient, a combination of two or multiple internal problems at the same time will affect your glands and hormones, and cause you to have an infectious disease.

Reasons why we have internal hair loss.

Systemic here means relating to a system within the body. [No organ or gland works on its own. It works as a part of the body's system. So, if one is affected then something else will be affected]

Anything that disrupts the normal hair cycle can cause hair loss, including medications. There is no medication that strengthens the immune system. So, with this in mind, the best offense is the best defense. You must take on the task of strengthening the body's entire system, rather than medicate it to death. True medications have their part, but I think we jump to the gun too quickly. A quote from my childhood says it best; "Conversation rules the Nation, so let's talk." I'll add this to it; "so, get the Education!"

In getting the education, how can you make certain you are being given the correct information? The best answer to this question is to study. Know your history of what worked in the past (like eating right), and add experience of good ole' wisdom. But some things you have to try and see if it works for you. With that said, I think you should try more of a Holistic approach before you "Go Med!" Medications have side effects, but a natural (Non-GMO) approach doesn't have side effects. You will either have an allergic reaction to these natural medicines or you will not. Usually there are more plants or herbs that can do the same thing, so just switch and try another.

To go too deep into physiologic or emotional stresses and endocrine imbalances (hormone disorders) would take us way left of this chapter's true focus and to what most people do already; Go Med! But we will mention a few things of concern. Our goal is to look more into strengthening what is already strong or weak and make **it** even stronger; your BODY! Your body is so incredible. It's designed to heal itself. The question is, when we have a problem, "Why isn't it healing?" There are a combination of things that can hinder repair of the body; if we focus only on the visual or irritant thing, our present focus maybe wrong. You always should ask why? So, let's look at the Why's. First, the fuel of the body. If you put the wrong fuel, or a fuel that has contaminants that are contrary to your motorized vehicle's needs, then it will not run smoothly, or it will break down quickly or even later. If someone puts sugar in your automobile's gas tank and your engine stops running, do you only focus on the engine? No, you examine the engine and trace it to the contaminants, sugar in your tank. (Today's Pesticides and Herbicides are two kinds of contaminants). You would principally have the same problems if you were to put water in your car's gas tank or where the oil pan goes. That's the point of this chapter—to put the healthier & right things in the body that will have a positive effect on your skin and hair. This will probably cause you to have a healthier life! And who doesn't want to have a healthy body in their life.

Here are just a few cases where your body goes through hormone changes. Hormonal disorders or changes can cause hair loss. I believe the key is counteracting through diet and supplements, to lessen the effects of those changes or to just understand what's happening. We should treat each hair loss situation with a curious eye of inspection and a critical thinking mind. We should be watching and examining each person, looking at what's happening in their life, assessing what they're eating, considering their known medical situations and what medications they are taking, and checking their family medical history for such conditions as iron deficiency or thyroid problems. If your family had them and your lifestyle and eating habits are similar, then you may have them now and don't know or you may develop them in the future.

Let's just quickly look at a couple of common hair loss occurrence, Iron deficiency, Menopause, and Pregnancy.

IRON DEFICIENCY

Iron deficiency is one of the most common deficiencies of the world. Most people don't know this. It affects about 25% of the people worldwide. Men and women are both affected by low iron. Men need more iron than women. It is an essential mineral in which the main component is red bloods cells and it delivers oxygen to the cells all over the body. Iron is hardly ever a deficiency that happens by itself. Normally when your iron is low you have a couple of other deficiencies along with it. Low levels of iron can cause constant hair shedding, even though you are treating the hair correctly. Shed strands of hair will normally be the length of your hair on your head. No matter how much you do conditioning treatments, it just keeps shedding. Relaxed hair just seems to shed even more. Most people don't know how to recognize their deficiency. *Vegetarians are more likely to have iron deficiency because of their meatless diet.* Here are some other symptoms:

- General fatigue

- Weakness

- Anemia

- Brittle nails

- Cold hands and feet

- Craving for ice

- Dizziness

- Glossy eyes

- Weakened immune system

- Impaired brain function

- Headaches

Iron deficiency is very treatable disorder, but you might need to have a life style change of your diet. Blackstrap molasses is a good source of iron. It's a high concentration of vitamins and minerals.

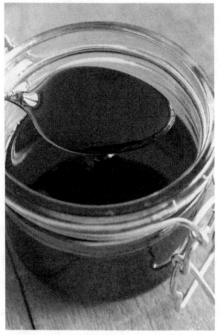

Blackstrap Molasses (above)

Spirulina is another good source for iron, and it is recommended for vegans because of its high iron content. Vitamin C is a good complementary supplement to iron because it helps your absorption of it.

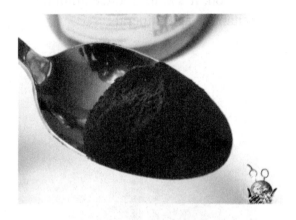

Spirulina is also called Pond scum. It's a natural "Blue-Green algae" powder that's rich in protein, iron, B-1, calcium and antioxidants. It can be considered one of the most potent nutrient sources. It is highly recommended for vegetarians, and is ideal during pregnancy and for building up of your immune system.

Spirulina is considered to match eggs per grams as a

protein source. It also helps with digestion of fats and proteins. Spirulina is excellent to help with increasing energy, eye health, and brain function. It also gives 26 times the amount of calcium than milk does.

By wellnessmama.com

Make sure you check the RDA *and use it correctly. Read reactions and allergies of Spirulina before using. (at back of book)*

MENOPAUSE

In the case of menopause, having knowledge is good, but combining that knowledge with a healthy diet will do more to lessen your hair loss. In menopause, your hair growth stage is shortened over time, but there are some foods that will strengthen your growth stage by supporting and lengthening your hair's growth cycle. There are certain things you can add in your diet that will strengthen and improve your skin, hair, and nails.

PREGNANCY

During pregnancy, there is an increase in hormones, which alters a woman's normal hair shedding cycle. Then after pregnancy the body works to return to the regular pattern of shedding 75-150 strands of hair per day. All the hair that a woman will shed during pregnancy may fall out all at once. This is not the entire head of hair, just the natural daily portion. A woman will still have much of her hair, if it is just after the pregnancy period. Therefore, women do not need to panic because the hair loss, but this is just temporary until the body balances back out.

The body should normalize within 6-12 months.

In this case, it's important to know what is actually happening with your body. Your estrogen and progesterone hormones go through sudden and dramatic increases These increases cause multiple changes with your body, from mood, weight gain, effects on the inside of the body and within the skin, hair & nails to say a few. You want to have a superb diet because you need to be in the best health possible to feed your baby. And if you are breast-feeding after, its best for you to maintain that diet until you finish breast-feeding your newly born sweetheart. I would even go in to say keep that good diet to teach your child how to eat. Be that good example and by being as healthy as possible you'll produce optimal nutrients for your hair and skin to grow at it's best. This

can cause you and your child to have the
best & healthy internal organ support. With
that said let's go even deeper than the skin.

Organs that Affect Your Hair & Skin

Now let's talk about what organs affect the
skin, hair and nails.

The Liver, Kidney, Adrenals,
Thyroid, Large & Small Intestines all
effect the hair and skin. Let's make this
more visible to your mind by giving you
more details.

Your liver is a major player on
your team of organs. It produces
energy to maintain the thousands
of functions performed by all
your body's cells. If your liver is
broken and not able to do its job
of breaking down toxins
efficiently and excreting wastes
through the proper channels, in

many cases those harmful materials will be expelled through the skin! As the deep layers of your skin become full of toxins, inflammation or skin errors develop in the form of:

- Acne
- Brown spots
- Dermatitis
- Eczema
- Painful rashes
- Psoriasis
- Red itchy rashes and more

Skin problems that continue to get worse could be a sign of a broken liver or future broken one. Most treatments for skin errors use creams, drugs or a combination of both to suppress the rash or whatever present issue is affecting the skin. *But that problem could be an immune system dysfunction. These strong* medicines *have side effects.* When your skin is treated with strong medications, toxins are pushed deeper into the body and this may cause health problems later on.

In dealing with the liver, with a hair view point, the focus should be on noticing the signs of the skin that give warning of a potential liver disorder. Disruptions of the skin can cause disruption of your hair growth cycle and can have a trickle down effect to hair loss. So it's best to look into getting the liver checked out when you see these signs. You can also reset your body by doing a full body or an organ cleanse; because your body can naturally, is some cases, heal itself. When you detox you tend to have more energy because of the lack of toxins in the body. It's also important to remember to strengthen and support your liver and immune system.

"Beware of Tylenol. Deadliest drug in America; kills more Livers than anything." By Dr. John Bergman

Let's look into the kidneys,

The kidneys are two bean-looking organs that, like the liver, help to eliminate waste from the blood in the form of urine. What we must see here is that the kidneys, like the liver get rid of waste from the body. And if they are not functioning properly it can and will come through your skin and disrupt it. Thus can cause and trickle down affect and aid in hair loss. Remember your body is a system that works with everything within your body.

> *"Aspirin a day; is the leading cause of Kidney Disease. Blood pressure drugs damage the kidneys also." By Dr. John Bergman*

Now let's look at the **Adrenal glands.** This can get a little tricky but you'll get it. Just remember that will have been talking about external and internal relationships the whole time. They can cause hair loss when they have a chronic fatigue syndrome, the fight or flight state.

Hair loss and weak immune system are two of the chronic inflammatory responses that adrenal fatigue causes.

"In many cases "Adrenals are chronically fatigue from Staten drugs." By Dr. John Bergman

Statin drugs are basically inhibitors. They slow down the production cholesterol in the liver.

Cholesterol is essential for the normal function of every cell in the body. With this said, its for you to relate that if you are on some statin drugs (inhibitors) for your walk of life, that this could be related to your hair loss problem.

The **Thyroid** is an organ that most of us know can indirectly affect your hair. But many don't know that if your Adrenal glands are constantly in a fatigue syndrome (revved up), the fight or flight state, it can result in the thyroid functioning poorly. And it will also appear as though you have a thyroid problem that causes you bad hair loss, but it's really your adrenals run hard for too long. The fight or flight state is basically when your body's adrenalin increase to fight and defend against a threat or to take flight and run away as fast as you can to escape and call the police! When your adrenal glands are in this state they use up the energy and cause your thyroids to perform at a low rate. The adrenals running high is only suppose to be temporary not constant for long periods of time. Just like if your car is ran in high gear all the time something within the car's system would break, malfunction or shut down. So now you can see if the adrenals are in a fatigue state, they lower the thyroid function. The low thyroid function then affects the hair. The thyroid stores and produces hormones that affect every organ in your body. Some of the symptoms of an overactive and underactive thyroid are:

- Autoimmune diseases
- Poor quality of hair and nails
- Hair loss
- Skin conditions such as acne

- Run down and tired
- Weight gain
- May feel "hyper"

The adrenals and the thyroid cannot run high or low at the same time. However, the behavior of the adrenals determines how the thyroid will act. If the adrenals are low, then you have a high functioning thyroid, and vice-versa.

"Thyroids are constantly weakened from being in a systemic inflammation state…Small and Large intestines are affected by all the commercially produced meats, antibiotics and all the glyphosates (herbicide) in our foods." By Dr. John Bergman

All these organs have some effect on the skin, when any one of them is malfunctioning let alone multiple ones. The skin is the largest organ of the body. The hair & nails are appendages (extensions) of the skin. So, whatever happens to the skin can affect the hair or even cause hair loss. If

118

you have medicine that states that it causes dehydration or affects the skin or nail in some manner, then it can cause hair loss, especially with people with chemically relaxed hair because it's in a weaker state, but can still be resilient. Many things or a combination of things can cause the body to become toxic in some manner causing hair loss to occur from the previously mentioned contaminants to the body:

- Tylenol
- Aspirin
- Statin drugs (inhibitors) Like-
    - Lipitor
    - Lescol
    - Altoprev
    - Pravachol
    - Crestor
    - Zocor

- Commercially produced meats
  - Fast-food meats
  - Cold cuts
  - GMO meats
- Antibiotics
- And Glyphosates (herbicide) in our foods.

Now let's get back to this chapter's main focus, to build up and strengthen the body's system. So, if you do things to strengthen these vital organs, feed them what they need, you create a perfect, or at least a better, environment. This environment will allow you to have and produce stronger Skin (organ), hair & nails and eliminate a lot of hair loss problems. I know it sounds like I'm telling you to go Vegan. You have to make that choice on your own, based on how much your hair and health means to you and how much of a part you want to play in living your life to the fullest. My focus is to make you think about adding positive things, but I have to tell you about both sides.

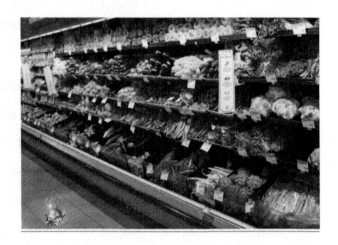

The optimal diet for skin and hair health

- Organic plant based diet (locally grown, seasonal foods)
- Healthy fats such as coconut oil and olive oil
- Fermented vegetables

- Probiotic supplements
- Juice vegetables
- Blend fruits
- Raw dairy
- Reduce Omega 6 and increase animal based Omega 3"

By Dr. John Bergman

Let's start getting stronger with building our gut up. An organic plant based diet, healthy fats, Fermented vegetables and more listed above, increase the health of the body's "Gut Flora" or also known as Gut bacteria, there's good & bad bacteria within the Gut Flora, but a healthy one is balanced. All the food mentioned to build and keep your Gut balanced or to bring it back from being unbalanced are all Non-GMO produced.

- WE need to build up our internal ecosystem, which helps with digesting food, assisting out immune system and producing nutrients for our body.

- Added a smoothie to you diet is a good way to add raw blended fruits
- One of my favorite probiotic supplements is "Green Vibrance, powder" by Vibrant Health. It also comes in capsule form.

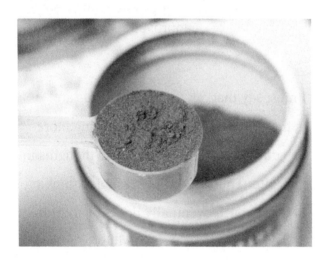

- Raw milk. I mention this for the baby factor because it contains beneficial nutrients for a new born's immune system that gives the baby's internal ecosystem a boost. I'm talking about from human to human tho. If you can't breast feed your baby, I would suggest thinking about supplementing in some Spirulina and Green Vibrance. Consult with your physician first for approval.

I must say that my theory and focus are getting people interested in focusing more on adding the positive foods and thoughts in their life. Thus by adding them and thinking of them you'll eventually do less bad. But here I want to tell you about the foods that studies say to reduce for better health. I think that's only fare. I want your knowledge to be well rounded as I mentioned before.

Reduce Omega 6 and **increase animal based Omega-3.**

- Some Omega 6 fats are necessary, but the Western diet gives us way more than we need. I personally find a Caribbean diet tends to be healthier, because it focuses on keeping with natural herbs, spices, fresh fish, unprocessed meats and mostly cooking at home. Omega 6 foods can have a MAJOR effect on the body by increasing inflammation. Here are some examples of Omega 6 foods:

1. *Sugar and High-Fructose Corn Syrup*
2. *Artificial Trans Fats*

3. *Vegetable and Seed Oils*
4. *Refined Carbohydrates*
   a. *White bread, White rice and etc (bleach products)*
   b. *Note: Refined carbohydrates are altered in some way or process, such as through industrial extraction, concentration, purification (bleaching) and enzymatic transformation.*
5. *Excessive Alcohol*
6. *Processed Meat*

We should be eating more Omega-3 rich foods, such as fatty fish. A balanced ratio of

Omega 6 to Omega-3 foods provides the body with anti-inflammatory benefits.

Omega-3 fatty acids have beneficial properties for your body such as enhancing the nervous system, vision and brain function. Think about this: 60% of the brain is made up of fats. *Algae, such as Spirulina, has high amounts of Omega-3's. Here are a few foods that are high in Omega-3s.*

- *Flaxseed*

- *Herring*

- *Mackerel*

- *Salmon*

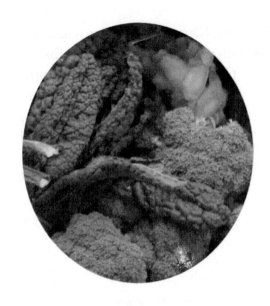

The Basics of Skin and Hair Health

"Dark Green leafy vegetables

Promote optimal function of natural detoxification systems

- Kale
- Spinach
- Dandelion greens
- Broccoli
- Chlorella"

By Dr. John Bergman

One way you can tell if you are naturally detoxing is that you go to the restroom 2-3 times a day for a bowel movement. In our fight to not have a toxic rich body is to detox. The body fights not to remain loaded with toxins. This is why if the liver and kidneys' are not doing their jobs, it's common to have skin problems.

- ○ Ex. If your colon is full of toxins. You might have dark blotches and acne on your cheeks. This is a tall tail sign to add more dark leafy vegetables and supplements (Green Vibrance) in your diet. And you might want to decrease on heavy meat at the same time. Your bowels should float not sink. If they sink keep increasing your green and decrease your meats. If you're on a lot of meds, please consult with a professional on how to periodically cleanse your body without putting yourself into a health risk situation. Find what works for you and your present health state.

- Note: If you are on a blood thinner, such as Warfarin, brand name: Coumadin, dark leafy vegetables and Green Vibrance (the Vitamin or foods with K2 in them) will be counter productive with your MEDS.

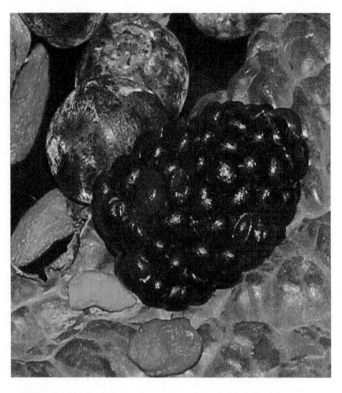

(The above picture is to focus on the Blackberries, Blueberries and store bought Goji berries)

<u>The Basics of Skin and Hair Health</u>

Antioxidant rich food

Help protect your body against for radicals

1. Goji berries
2. Wild blueberries
3. Dark chocolate
4. Pecans
5. Artichoke
6. Elderberries
7. Blackberries
8. Kidney beans

Let's look into what's an Antioxidant?

"A substance that inhibits oxidation, especially one used to counteract the deterioration of stored food products. Vitamin C or E helps to reduce oxidation. They are also used in anti-aging creams and for healing of the skin.

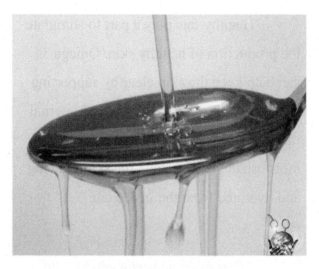

(Olive Oil in above image)

<u>The Basics of Skin and Hair Health</u>

Healthy fats

Supports healthy hormone production and supports skin regeneration

1. Omega 3
2. Coconut oil
3. Olive oil
4. Organic grass-fed butter

By Dr. John Bergman

Healthy fats play a part to stimulate the production of healthy skin. Omega 3s can help keep the skin clear by supporting the fight against both external and internal inflammation. And are perfect for moisturizing and keeping the skin glowing and hydrated from the inside out.

"Fats exert powerful effects within the body.
We need adequate fat to support metabolism, cell signaling, the health of various body tissues, immunity, hormone production, and the absorption of many nutrients (such as vitamins A and D).
Having enough fat will also help keep you feeling full between meals. Healthy fats have been shown to offer the following benefits.

Average evidence
- *Prevent cancers*
- *Preserve memory*
- *Preserve eye health*

- *Reduce incidence of aggressive behavior*
- *Reduce ADHD and ADD symptoms"*

For more info:
http://www.precisionnutrition.com/all-about-healthy-fats

The Basics of Skin and Hair Health

- Help promote growth of beneficial bacteria, supports healthy immune function
- Help increase vitamin B, omega 3, digestive enzyme, and lactase/lactic acid
     1. Kefir (fermented milk)
     2. Kombucha
     3. Sauerkraut
     4. Pickles
     5. Miso
     6. Kimchi

Fermented foods are good for healing the Gut and

having a healthy "Gut Flora." If you heal the gut you heal the immune system. Remember "AA" hair loss is an immune system disorder. *By Dr. John Bergman*

An impaired gut flora has been connected with a host of inflammatory and autoimmune conditions. Hair loss is one of those indirect connected issues. Gut flora is also called Gut bacteria, which is a healthy balance of "Good & Bad" bacteria inside your belly. I say "good" before bad because it should be the greater of the two. In my studies, I found that it's very hard to get sick when your good bacteria are higher than your bad bacteria. This simply means you have a strong immune system. The University School of Medicine has found that there is a relationship between an unbalanced gut bacteria and multiple sclerosis (MS). People with an unbalanced gut bacteria have also been found to have a widespread of symptoms including bloating, gas, cramps, inflammatory bowel disease (IBD), fatigue, food sensitivities, sleeplessness and skin problems as eczema & psoriasis. Another problem that can arise is from your gut being out of balance, a condition called Leaky Gut Syndrome, where particles of undigested food and toxins enter the blood stream. So not only does having a healthy gut improve your skin health & vibrancy, it also can keep you out of the hospital. So skin errors can be directly and indirectly related to health issues that are deeper than the skin.

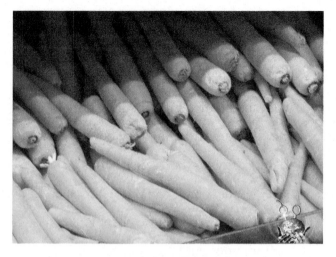

The Basics of Skin and Hair Health

Carotenoids

Two categories carotene and xanthophils

1. Carrots
2. Sweet potatoes
3. Kale
4. Spinach
5. Astaxanthin (from marine algae; like Spirulina)

By Dr. John Bergman

One of these is usually one of the main ingredients in juicing and helps keep a your skin in good health. By eating foods that contain carotenoids, people gain protective health benefits such as cancer-fighting abilities and improved vision. The vitamin A in carotenoids also aids normal growth and development. By strengthening the immune system it indirectly helps in cardiovascular disease prevention. As you go further in this chapter you will start to understand this quote I have at the beginning: *"Let food be thy medicine and medicine be thy food."*

As you can see once again, by adding the benefits of eating right, you strengthen your immune system and it helps you fight against inflammation that could be associated to your skin and hair loss.

<u>Feed your skin and hair from the outside</u>

1. Organic Shea butter
2. Cocoa butter
3. Virgin coconut oil
4. Jojoba oil
5. Murumuru butter
6. Palm oil
7. Aloe vera juice

By Dr. John Bergman

These are plants above are great for topical use. And most are used in the cosmetology and skin care industries. If you take the time to not only listen to the marketing keys words, but also look into the ingredient labels. Shea butter, jojoba oil, Aloe Vera and different forms of the coconut; such as coconut butter, coconut oil and coconut water, are commonly use in products.

- *Shea Butter is rich in vitamins A, E and F. It gives protection from the sun and reduces inflammation. Thus, it helps to improve the skin & hair.*
- *Aloe vera has a host of medical claims of the benefits concerning it. Some are back up by scientific studies and some are not.*
- Jojoba oil and the various form of the coconut are great moisturizers and good for hydration as well.

Vitamin D

Vitamin D deficiency is linked to:

1. Digestive disorders
2. Skeletal disorders including osteoporosis
3. Depression, mental disorders
4. Neurodevelopmental disorders (Autism)
5. Brain dysfunction, dementia and Alzheimer's
6. Chronis infection
7. Cardiovascular disease
8. All types of cancer
9. Autoimmune diseases
10. Premature aging

By Dr. John Bergman

Vitamin D deficiency is related to "AA" (Alopecia Areata), hair loss, and virtually every type of cancer. Certain times of year, during the flu season, you need to take Vitamin D supplements for the lack of available sunlight. The sun is the best way to absorb and optimize your body's Vitamin D needs. Adults should take about 5,000-8,000 IUs per day. If you become sick, you can increase them to about 6 times the average for at least the first week.

Vitamin K2 is essential for proper utilization of vitamin D. Some good sources of vitamin K2 are Grass-fed organic animal products (eggs, butter and dairy), fermented foods and certain cheeses (Brie, Gouda)

By Dr. John Bergman

Vitamin K2 is found mainly in green leaves and essential for the blood-clotting process. Remember if you're on blood thinners beware of K2, and consult with your doctor because they could be counter productive with your medications.

"L-Carnitine plays a key role in the intramitochondrial transport of fatty acids for beta-oxidation and thus serves important functions in energy metabolism. Here, we have tested the hypothesis that L-Carnitine, a frequently employed dietary supplement, may also stimulate hair growth by increasing energy supply to the massively proliferating and energy-consuming anagen hair matrix."

"Our findings suggest that L-Carnitine stimulates human scalp hair growth by up regulation of proliferation and down regulation of apoptosis in follicle keratinocytes in vitro."

By Experimental Dermatology

L-Carnitine is another great ingredient that enhances the growth of your hair strand. In more simply words, L-Carnitine increases the ability for the hair to grow and slows down the death, (it increases the life cycle of your hair). It helps it to grow **Longer and Stronger**! Now, who

144

doesn't want their hair to grow like that. This part of my book can be taken to the grocery store to help you shop for good food to add to your diet. Here's a list from Dr. John Bergman on foods that are good sources of L-Carnitine. My favorites are in **bold**:

- ***Red meat (highest source) (organic is recommended)***
- ***Seafood***
- ***Chicken***
- *Dairy (raw dairy)*
- *Nuts*
- *Seeds*
- *Artichokes*
- ***Asparagus***
- ***Broccoli***
- *Brussels sprout*
- ***Collard greens***
- *Garlic*
- *Mustard greens*

Plants for Hair Health

Here are some plants that I learned about from Dr. John Bergman. Some I knew of and some I didn't. Most of these plants are to be applied topically, on top of the skin.

- Onion juice
- Asiasari Radix
- Gingko Biloba
- Hibiscus leaf
- Peppermint oil
- Sophora Flavescens
- Green tea
- Grape Seed extract
- Turmeric

By Dr. John Bergman

Onion juice

"This study was designed to test the effectiveness of topical crude onion juice in the treatment of patchy Alopecia Areata...

- ***Re-growth of Terminal coarse hairs*** *started after two weeks of treatment with crude onion juice.*
- *At four weeks, hair re-growth was seen in 73.9% of patients*

- *At 6 weeks, the hair re-growth was observed 86.9%*

  By Journal of Dermatology

In this treatment you probably want to use a juicer and place it in a glass container with a few pedals in the jar of juice for application purposes, or you can find a different method that works for you. I noticed that the smell reduces after about 20min, and continues to decrease as the day goes on. You will probably notice it more than others. When I tried it no one knew until I told them, two weeks into my 4 weeks trial of this treatment. I tried to use it as I thought that the average person might. I used it for the first 5 days straight. Then I did it every other day. I even missed at least 2 days every now and then on purpose. At the end I let my hair grow and didn't shave it. To my surprise a few of my clients and family members said "Hey some of your hair came back!" I just laughed and said "You can tell?", with a high pitched voice of joy. This was because all of them didn't know about the treatment. And yes it did grow back some. Plus I wasn't consistent with my applications. I only applied it once a day. Some of the recommendations said to apply 2-3 times a day. I found this out after I started and didn't want to change my routine of my treatment. I plan on trying this again for research purposes or one of the of the others that you're read about after this. Now, I do have to say most of the women that I told of the treatment, were Not willing to try it for the most part of two reasons. One was because of the fear of smelling like onions juice; even though I told them no one knew I had been using it for a few weeks.

The second was, they were worried about how they would style their hair doing the process of the 6-8 weeks that I recommended to test it out. I thought, Vanity, Vanity, there are so many slaves to Vanity! As I smile at their response of, "I don't think I can do that."

Asiasari Radix

"We examined the effects of 45 extracts that have been traditionally used for treating hair loss in oriental medicine in order to Identify potential stimulants of hair growth."

*Among the tested plants extract, the extract of Asiasari **Radix showed the most potent hair growth stimulation...***"

> By Journal of Dermatology Science

Gingko Biloba

"Gingko Biloba (GBE) showed a promoting effect on the hair growth. GBE had the

inhibitory effects on blood platelet aggregation, thrombin activity and fibrinolysis."

*"These results suggest that GBE **promote the hair regrowth** and could be used as a hair tonic."*

By Yakugako Zasshi of Journal of the Pharmaceutical Society of Japan

Hibiscus Leaf Extract

"...extract of leaves and flowers of Hibiscus Rosa-sinensis was evaluated for its potential on hair growth by in vivo and vitro methods."

*"From the study it is conclude that the leaf extract, when compared to flower extract, **exhibits more potency on hair growth**."*

By Journal of Ethno pharmacology

Hibiscus leaf extract works in vivo method (within the natural setting) and in vitro method (within a lab or in a controlled environment) also. Can be used topically.

Peppermint Oil

"These results suggest that Peppermint Oil **induces a rapid anagen stage** *(the hair growth stage) and could be used for a practical agent for hair growth without change of body weight gain and food efficiency."*

By Toxicology Research

Peppermint oil helps accelerate hair growth during the growth stage of the hair cycle. And can be used in professional and homemade shampoos.

Sophora Flavescens

"In search of natural extract for hair growth, we found that the extract of dried root of Sophora Flavescens has **outstanding** *hair growth promoting effect."*

By Zeitschrift fur Naturforschung C, Journal of Biosciences

Grape Seed Extract

*"For the purpose of discovering natural products which possess hair growth activity, we examined about 1000 kinds of plant extracts concerning growth-promoting activity with respect to hair follicle cells. After an extensive search, we discovered that proanthocyanidins extracted from grape **seed promote proliferation of hair cells**..."*

By Acta Dermato-Venerologica, Journal of Clinical and Experimental Research

Grape Seed Extract takes dormant cells and helps them to work better.

By Dr. John Bergman

Curcumin for All skin disorders

"Turmeric (Curcuma Longa), a commonly used spice throughout the world, has been shown to exhibit anti-inflammatory, antimicrobial, antioxidant, and anti-neoplastic properties. Growing evidence shows that an active component of turmeric, curcumin, may be used medically to treat a variety of dermatologic disease."

"Skin conditions examined include acne, alopecia, atopic dermatitis, facial photoaging, oral lichen planus, pruritus psoriasis, radiodermatitis, and vitiligo... Overall, there is early evidence that turmeric/curcumin products and supplements, both oral and topical, may provide therapeutic benefits for skin health."

By Phytotherapy Research

Turmeric is good for all skin ailments. **By Dr. John Bergman**

Coconut Oil for Health

1. *Rich in antioxidants*

153

2. *Antiviral*
3. *Antifungal*
4. *Antibacterial*
5. *Improves scalp health*
6. *Fights infections and fungi*
7. *Supports hair growth*
8. *Adds volume and shine*

Great for scalp health, especially after toxic scalp exposure.

By Dr. John Bergman

These are the questions I asked my clients with dry scalp issues. Some of them went to the physician and found out about an unknown health issue through the signs and questions I asked. Now answer them for yourself. Then look back through this chapter and create: a new grocery list, things to eat or avoid when eating out, what vitamins to add, is there a more holistic approach to my problem, and last maybe I need to see a couple of professionals because I have signs that are deeper than the skin. One thing I want you to know. It's not that you change over night, but It's more important that you keep it moving in spite of the mistakes along the way! It took me three times to do a 30 day cleanse and get it 80% correct. I still struggle now with things, but I feel so much better. I'm not where I use to be, BUT I AM STRONGER THAN I WAS!

- "What do you eat?
  - Any fruits and vegetables regularly?
- Are you on any Meds?
  - If so, do any of your Meds affect the skin, hair or nails?
- Do you have any health problems with you or in your family involving the Liver, Kidneys, Adrenals, Thyroid or Large & Small intestines?

Grocery List for Food and Supplements

Create your own list of healthy groceries and supplements to enhance your body and life. I hope this chapter gets you started on making better choices, even if it's just a little bit at a time. What's most important is that you Start!

6

Conclusion

In understanding the fundamentals to prevent hair damage, it was imperative to first learn to identify internal hair loss and external hair breakage. Then examine the various contributing factors for each. You can damage your hair externally, which is the lighter of the two, regardless of the immediate result that may appear flawed. Secondly, you can also damage your hair internally, which is more detrimental to not only the hair strand, but the systems of your body, your health and life itself. **So, remember what you put in the body, food, medicine and supplements, can cause internal damage as well.**

I believe respect is birth out of the knowledge we have about someone or something. So, base on this thought, I wanted you to meet your hair and skin. They are of the same family, "Integumentary system" is their maiden name. They have an intimate relationship. Each has their own characteristics but they are still connected. I wanted you to see them in your mind, then remind you that they are brothers and sisters of the same family. Therefore, respect the relationship when you are performing services no matter how simple that service is.

In building your knowledge of your hair and then building an intimate relationship with it, you will understand the first half of this quote:" **Know your Hair, Know your Product**". that I truly believe in this quote. Equally important is knowing your product. I have seen different problems that are common and some not so common problems that people may not know about the products they are using. This is one chapter that you should refer to and read over multiple times until you become familiar with the choice of products that you pick. Understanding the products, you use and what they do, would increase your ability to work more effectively and get the result you desire. Now, by knowing your hair and understanding your product you can respect the Hair to Product relationship. Do your best not to violate the intimacy of your hair and skin connection. In addition, I wanted you to be more careful about the marketing ads that you hear and act upon. Remember marketing is a business tool. They only have to use a seed of truth and the rest could be the dream. A little bit of truth and a lot of fantasy is the skill of marketing. My advice to you, go and see a professional and get a factual advice. Even if you are on a budget, you can find a professional that can fit your budget.

I made the word hydration a ubiquitous term used throughout this book. It is my way of programming your mind to always keep water as a key for your internal and external. You should always be on the hair defense to maintain healthy at all cost. **Dehydration is Detrimental. Keeping Hydration is Essential! Water is LIFE, even with your Hair!**

In our efforts to prevent baldness, remember when something bad happened in your life, and how focusing on that negative gave it strength in your life. In much the same way focusing on baldness sometimes creates a negative sequel of events that makes it appear to increase your baldness. I think we focus on the negative views too much. If our eyes are only focusing on the negative, our mindset is negative. I had an Epiphany in my life where I stop looking at the glass as half empty, and started looking at it as half full. Though I have the same issues and problems it was my mindset that change things. My outlook went from negative to positive. Then better things happen for me. I became a happier person, in my heart and mind. Focus on healthy hair and not on the negative of unhealthy hair. I would wager that you will see better results.

There are some things that I have mentioned to beware of, but let's take a more positive approach and zone in on the good things that we can do for your hair and their benefits. After reading the last chapter your eyes should be open bit more. You should know to beware of putting contaminants in your body. Yet, your main focus should be building up your endocrine system, immune system, Gut Flora, and the other systems of your body by eating for hydration and nutrition. If you focus on putting good things in your body then it can heal itself most of the time.. Only "Go MED" when it's a must. You learn about seeking professionals for advice from nutrition, to hair services, health issues by paying attention to the signs that your body is telling you: Remember know your hair know your product!

I wrote this book to help you to have an open mind and to increase understanding, to impart some of my wisdom from over thirty years in the hair business. Help you to recognize and learn from past mistakes and how to correct it or go see a professional. It's okay to do-it-yourself but in acquire the knowledge and check the facts. Always check with a professional when things become risky, so you don't end up as a famous YouTube video. I want you to leave this book empowered, and with a joyous heart to start doing things better and with a sense that is okay to make a *little* mistakes along the way to living a better and more for fulfilled life!

Appendix

Detox

Note: These are only suggestions. Referred to your physician before beginning. Cleanse the entire body for 30 days (wait 30 days before detoxing for another 30 days).

During detox:

1. Take detox programs. (I like Dual Action Cleanse pills), but there are a variety of systems you can use. Consult with a doctor for one that works with you. Check your local health food store for more options to suit you.)

2. Do not eat beef.

3. Do not eat pork.

4. Do not eat fried foods.

5. Eat something green every day. This should be a vegetable.

6. Drink 32 ounces of water by noon and 32 ounces of water by bedtime.

7. Eat, at least once, half a fruit per day as a meal.

8. Eat every three hours, or five meals a day. First meal should begin between 7:00 a.m.–8:00 a.m. as a general practice (adjust according to your work schedule).

9. Give yourself one or two cheat meals per week, but this meal must be

eaten by 1:00 p.m. or 2:00 p.m. (your third meal).

10. Give yourself at least a week to prepare before starting the detox. In preparation, find different restaurants and places to eat last minute if you forget to prepare your meals.

Cautions of Spirulina

There are three known categories cautions related to spirulina: reactions, diarrhea and stomach upset, and heavy metal poisoning.

Reactions and Allergies
People can be allergic to almost anything on the planet...Foods, medications, animal dander, plant pollen and many other substances can cause reactions and allergies, including spirulina.

Some people have mild reactions to spirulina. These allergic reactions may include a rash or skin discomfort. Rarely, severe reactions may occur. These include hives, difficult breathing, and asthma-like symptoms. If you've taken spirulina and have trouble breathing, you may be severely allergic and need medical attention. Stop taking spirulina and see a physician immediately. Usually mild allergy symptoms go away on their own after people stop taking spirulina.

Diarrhea and Stomach Upset

A most unpleasant reaction to spirulina is the danger of stomach upset, specifically, diarrhea. Usually this happens when people take too much spirulina. Always follow label and package directions carefully, and never exceed the recommended dose. Each product is manufactured differently, so one brand's dose may be different from another. When changing product brands, reread the label to ensure you're taking spirulina supplements according to package directions.

If stomach cramps and diarrhea occur, stop taking spirulina. Symptoms should pass within a short period of time once you stop taking spirulina supplements.

Heavy Metal Poisoning

By far the most frequently cited danger of spirulina is heavy metal toxicity or poisoning. How does a blue green algae poison someone? The answer lies in where the algae was grown and in how it is harvested. Spirulina is an algae, and algae grows on lakes, ponds and in man-made ponds. If the water it's grown in contains heavy metals such as mercury or lead, the little spirulina algae will absorb the metals. Then when they are harvested and dried into a supplement, the metals remain inside the supplement.

Fortunately, heavy metal toxicity from spirulina is very rare. When purchasing supplements, quality brands do make a difference. Many name brands have testing laboratories and provide test results to the general public. If you're concerned about heavy metals infesting your spirulina supplement, contact the manufacturer and ask if the supplement has been tested. Ask for a copy of the test results. If you follow the label directions and take only as much as is recommended, you should avoid contamination from heavy metals.

Spirulina Precautions

Spirulina is generally a safe supplement for the majority of people. Yes, allergies and reactions can occur, but allergies occur with common foods, too, such as dairy products or peanuts. Heavy metal poisoning from spirulina is uncommon. To be on the safe side, pregnant and nursing women should avoid taking spirulina supplements, since unborn babies and infants are at high risk for brain and nervous system damage if exposed to heavy metal toxins. Never harvest spirulina or algae in the wild. It may be contaminated. Without the proper testing equipment, you have no way of knowing if the algae has picked up bacteria or metal contaminants. Just because a body of water looks clean doesn't mean it is free from heavy metal poisons.

Spirulina can be a great dietary supplement. Use common sense, discontinue use if any side effects occur, and choose high quality supplements to be safe.

http://vitamins.lovetoknow.com/Danger_of_Spirulina

Tips

Hairstylists can be the first to know that your body is out of balance. Everything is in your hair. It can tell you everything. For example, if you have taken drugs it can show in inches of hair growth for each year. You can multi-bleach to clear signs of your history, but this will not clear beneath the scalp. You can also tell that your body might be low in iron if your hair falls out and if you are often tired and crave ice.

Do home pH test when you have unexplained hair loss. It could be a sign that something deeper is the real issue, like unknown sick is at hand.
Litmus paper for testing your body's pH at home

- The human body should be slightly alkaline at 7.4 ph.

- Diseases and cancer can't survive in an oxygen-rich alkaline state. You can't get sick if your good bacteria is higher than your bad bacteria. If your good bacteria is higher, then you're in oxygen-rich alkaline state. If your bad bacteria is higher, you're in an oxygen-deficient acidic state. (From "Monitoring your body's pH levels" on *Altered States*, http://altered-states.net/barry/update178/.)

  - Use the litmus paper test to test to see what your pH is; [red would indicate acidity, and blue would indicate alkaline.]

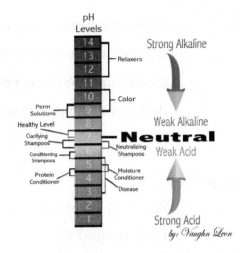

See the end of chapter 4 for large view.

How to Do a Scalp Detox

- o   Part head into 4 sections; no dandruff lift.

- o   Apply Black Carbon shampoo containing apple cider vinegar with a needle-nose application bottle. Then base entire scalp.

- o   Massage in for 1–3 minutes.

- o   Place head under dryer with a plastic cap for 10–15 minutes.

- Remove cap and add water to saturate and shampoo with present shampoo on scalp. Add more shampoo if needed.

Scalp Detox Plus

- Part head into 4 sections.
- Do a dandruff lift.
- Apply Black Carbon shampoo containing apple cider vinegar with a needle-nose application bottle. Then base entire scalp.
- Massage in for 1–3 minutes.
- Place under dryer with a plastic cap for 10–15 minutes.
- Remove cap and add water to saturate and shampoo with present shampoo on scalp. Add more shampoo if needed.

Hydrating Scalp Treatment

This is to be done after the hair has been shampooed and conditioned. Apply a light oil on scalp while the scalp is still damp. Liquid oil is harder to control when placing on the scalp; you might want to use solidified oil. Some great oils for your scalp are

- o Jojoba, Coconut and Olive oil are great oil for a dry dehydrated scalp. These oils are also good for fighting against the dry scalp of Psoriasis.

    Next, apply setting agents or leave-in conditioners. Let the oil dry into the scalp to prevent dryness and dehydration.

This procedure works because of the understanding that the skin breathes. When the skin is wet, it opens. This is the best time to apply moisture to counter dehydration. Note: you also can perform this after bathing so that you don't have to use a lotion. Apply oil to scalp after rinsing, then towel-dry.

Reading the Signs

You should develop your knowledge of the signs of the body. (I could write a book on this alone.) Here are a few signs that may lead you in the right direction as to whom to see or which area to check. Monitor these areas and have your professional physician check them out for any problems:

- Dark spots and acne on cheeks most likely means you need to cleanse your colon.

- Dry lips are a sign of body dehydration
- Thinning hair, swollen glands, weight loss, and glossy eyes could indicate thyroid problems.
- Dark spots in the middle of the foot sole point to kidney problems.
- Dehydrated skin and a flaky and dehydrated scalp may be a sign of lupus.
- Large scalp flakes indicate scalp bacteria.
- Small to large, greasy, yellow flakes and bald spots of about a quarter of the time are symptoms of a dandruff issue.

Circle of Professionals

- **Professional hairstylist:** Considered your general hair doctor.

- **Dermatologist:** Treats diseases, in the widest sense, and some cosmetic problems of the skin, scalp, hair, and nails.

- **Endocrinologist:** A physician who specializes in the management of hormone conditions.

- **General physician:** A medical doctor who treats acute and chronic illnesses and provides preventive care and health education to patients.

- **Holistic health doctor:** A doctor who may use all forms of health care, from conventional medication to alternative therapies, to treat a patient. The treatment plan may involve drugs to relieve symptoms, but also lifestyle modifications to

help prevent problems from
recurring.

○ **Trichologist:** A specialized hair loss
doctor. Trichology is the branch of
medical and cosmetic study and
practice concerned with the hair and
scalp. Another definition is the study
of hair and its diseases and how they
relate to the scalp.

Consultation questions

When was your last chemical?

What type was it?

Color

- ○ Permanent
  - Opaque
  - Translucent
- ○ Demi-permanent
  - Opaque

- Translucent
  - Semi/ rinse
    - Direct dye or not

According to the length...

Every 6-8 inches is roughly equal to a year

Ask how long since your color was applied to the length of the hair.

Ex. 20 in hair. Have you had a color within the last 3.5yrs

Bleach

Relaxer

Sodium hydroxide

- Mild
- Medium
- Coarse

Calcium (Guanidine) hydroxide

Did you get irritated

- Did you get based?

Did the relaxer go far down the hair shaft?

Have you flat iron your new growth recently?

 o   This could give you a
     false reading of where
     to apply relaxer

Scalp problems

What shampoo do you use?

How long do you wait between shampoos?

Did you scalp change soon after a chemical treatment?

So you have any skin disorders?

What do you eat?

Any fruits and vegetables regularly?

Are you on any Meds?

If so, do any of your Meds affect the skin, hair or nails?

Do you have any health problems with you or in your family involving the Liver, Kidneys,

Adrenals, Thyroid or Large & Small intestines?

References

1. Bobby J. Hunt, Orlando Florida
2. Dr. John Bergman DC, 18582 Beach Blvd, Huntington Beach, CA 92648
   a. https://www.youtube.com/watch?v=F1rxW9IzYrA&feature=youtu.be
   b. https://www.youtube.com/watch?v=xJa0X7J1lm4
   c. https://www.youtube.com/watch?v=rkumoDg8Zr8&t=374s
3. Lisa Akbari of World Trichology Institute, Southwest Tennessee Community College
   a. Trichology 101
4. http://www.hormone.org/contact-a-health-professional/what-is-an-endocrinologist
5. http://www.englishdermatology.com/library/4215/WhatisaDermatologist.html
6. https://www.google.com/webhp?sourceid=chrome-instant&ion=1&espv=2&ie=UTF-

8#q=hair%20follicle%20definition

7. http://encyclopedia.thefreedictionary.
com/Dermal+papillae

8. http://www.thefreedictionary.com/pa
pillary

9. https://www.google.com/webhp?sour
ceid=chrome-
instant&ion=1&espv=2&ie=UTF-
8#q=hair%20root%20define

10. http://www.dailyfinance.com/2013/1
1/21/foods-give-up-avoid-eating-
gmo/#!slide=1585543

11. http://naturalsociety.com/gmo-fed-
hamsters-become-infertile-have-
stunted-growth/#ixzz48xl5c9gC

12. http://naturalsociety.com/gmo-fed-
hamsters-become-infertile-have-
stunted-growth/#ixzz48xk07L5i

13. http://www.worldhairresearch.com/?
p=563#more-563

14. http://www.englishdermatology.com/
library/4215/WhatisaDermatologist.h
tml

15. http://altered-
states.net/barry/update178/

16. https://www.google.com/search?q=gl
    yphosate+define&oq=glyphosate+de
    fine&aqs=chrome..69i57j0.15127j0j
    7&sourceid=chrome&ie=UTF-
    8#safe=strict&q=statin+drugs+define
    d

17. https://www.google.com/search?q=s
    ystemic+inflammation+definition&o
    q=systemic+inflammation&aqs=chro
    me.2.69i57j0l5.4387j0j8&sourceid=c
    hrome&ie=UTF-8

18. www.naturalgirlsrock.com/blogs/.../1
    2212729-how-to-balance-**ph**-in-
    hair-naturally

19. http://obgyn.ucla.edu/fibroids

20. http://www.mayoclinic.org/diseases-
    conditions/uterine-
    fibroids/symptoms-causes/dxc-
    20212514

21. http://www.livestrong.com/article/44
    9516-iron-deficiency-and-blackstrap-
    molasses/

22. https://authoritynutrition.com/vitami
    n-d-deficiency-symptoms/

23. http://www.medicalnewstoday.com/a

rticles/14417.php

24. http://www.healthyhairplus.com/scal
p-oil-best-for-scalp-psoriasis-
s/4180.htm